Acclaim for
DON'T FORGET TO BREATHE

"Don't Forget to Breathe reminded me of my dad's advice: Steer into the skid. Shonda Moralis is amazing. She knows that balance doesn't come from a magic eraser that leaves you *ohm*ing in some silent, gardenia-scented space; it comes from paying attention to the chaos and clutter, to what's happening, to what matters. Plus, she lets you meditate while you're drinking coffee, so there's that, too."

—CATHERINE NEWMAN, author of *Waiting for Birdy*
and *Catastrophic Happiness*

"This book is what we all need. Apply these practices and start being present in your busy life—and find joy."

—LISA DRUXMAN, founder of FIT4MOM

"We all need that friend who believes in us and stands with us as we pursue our dreams. In *Don't Forget to Breathe* Shonda is that priceless friend. With powerful, yet gentle words she reminds us of the necessity of balance, helps us examine our dreams, and inspires us to breathe in the midst of life."

—RACHEL MARIE MARTIN, author of
The Brave Art of Motherhood

"Don't Forget to Breathe beautifully captures the importance of self-compassion for all women. Rather than adding one more thing to our to do lists, Moralis helps us cultivate a wise and powerful way of being as we move through each moment of our day."

—SHAUNA SHAPIRO, PhD, professor of cou~~~~~~
and author of *Good M(*

Also by Shonda Moralis

Breathe, Mama, Breathe:
5-Minute Mindfulness for Busy Moms

DON'T FORGET TO
Breathe

5-Minute Mindfulness for Busy Women

Shonda Moralis, MSW, LCSW

Author of *Breathe, Mama, Breathe*

THE EXPERIMENT

NEW YORK

*To Mom and Anika, my two most
beloved quietly powerful women.*

*And to Dad, Erik, and Ben, the strong
men who empower us to flourish.*

*A single breath is an instant
perspective changer.*
—Leah Weiss

CONTENTS

CHAPTER 2
Becoming Mindful Breaks 123

CHAPTER 3
Balance Mindful Breaks 205

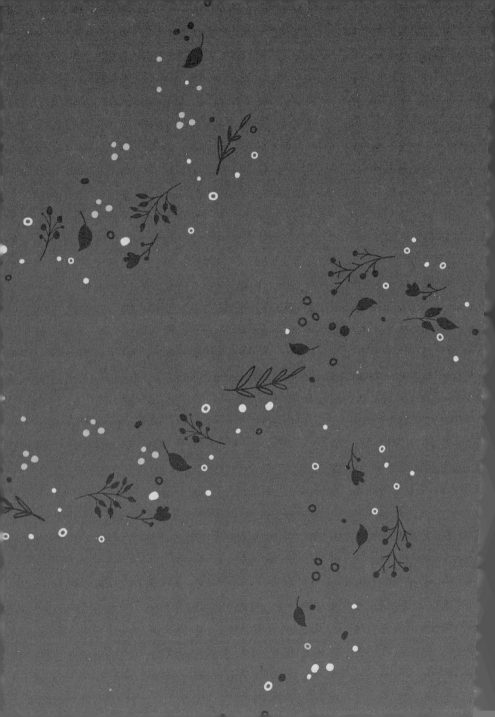

INTRODUCTION

Ditch the Stress without Losing Your Edge

When you quiet the mind and give it one thing to focus on, you quiet your body. When you quiet your body, you quiet your mind. When the mind and body are quiet, there is synergy that feeds pure performance.

—George Mumford

"There is never enough time in the day."

"I am spread so thin, no one receives my best. The guilt is constant and overwhelming."

"I'm not even sure who I am or what I enjoy."

"At the end of the day, there is nothing left for me—no energy, no time, no motivation."

"Work–life balance? What balance?"

Whoa. Heavy. I feel exhausted even typing those words onto the page and can imagine the effects of internalizing this dismal inner soliloquy day after day. Many of us do, whether or not we fully recognize it. And simply because everyone else looks like they are thriving, it doesn't mean they aren't struggling desperately on the inside. You thought it was just you? Not a chance. Welcome to the club.

When teaching mindfulness to women of all ages, in all types of careers, and in various phases of life, I repeatedly hear: We are stressed, overwhelmed, and time starved. Each of us hops onto the hamster wheel of busyness each morning, sprinting nonstop until we crash into bed in the evening—either falling fast asleep or grappling with insomnia—only to wake up the next morning and do it all over again. What work–life balance? Indeed.

Thankfully, life needn't feel so chaotic and overwhelming. Imagine I could offer you an all-natural prescription designed to induce a calmer, healthier sense of balance that will fill your days with sustained energy and an adequate amount of space to breathe. It is free and legal, generates no negative side effects, requires very little time, and is beneficial to your overall health. You in?

Research indicates that with regular mindfulness practice we can change the feel of the pace of our days from frantic and urgent to calm and efficient while also enhancing our health, productivity, and general well-being—no physician's prescription required. And all it takes is five minutes a day. Regardless of how busy our lives are, we can all carve out five minutes—I am convinced of it. I know; it sounds too good, too easy, too simple to be true.

I, too, was once skeptical of the seemingly counterintuitive ability to slow down yet accomplish more. As a recovering perfectionist, I have firsthand knowledge of the type A, workaholic-leaning buzz that comes from checking things off the beloved to-do list. I appreciate the palpable fear of losing one's edge, the apprehension that pausing for five entire minutes a day might precipitate the loss of precious creative momentum. Not to mention, I once thought, *Who in the world has time?* In his bestselling book

Tools of Titans: The Tactics, Routines, and Habits of Billionaires, Icons, and World-Class Performers, author Tim Ferriss shares replicable performance tips from dozens of highly successful people, and guess what? *Eighty percent* of the world-class performers interviewed in his book practice mindfulness, as does Ferriss himself. Whether this statistic is causal or correlational, it is certainly significant and not at all surprising. "Done consistently, my reward for meditating is getting thirty to fifty percent more done in a day with fifty percent less stress," Ferriss writes, echoing my own experience.

As you'll see, there are numerous reasons Arianna Huffington, Oprah, and Eileen Fisher meditate daily and regularly espouse its virtues and the direct influence it's had on their success—and subsequently share it with their respective teams. These women all recognize that the most effective outward growth and achievement originate from mindful insight, calmness, and self-awareness.

We may not be able to control all that life tosses our way, but we *can* adjust our perspective and automatic reaction to it. Mindfulness practice enables us to be more efficient, productive, and innovative without burnout or exhaustion. It teaches us how to be more in control of our responses in stressful situations rather than reacting without thinking. And, perhaps best of all, it allows us to more readily notice and savor the good that is already present in our lives.

Within these pages you will find an antidote to the ubiquitous instances of stress, overwhelm, and time starvation, with dozens of brief and evidence-based practices called mindful breaks. They are opportunities and reminders throughout the day to bring attention to what is happening *as it is happening* instead of operating on automatic pilot. We can take a mindful break at any time—when drinking coffee, while commuting to work, in the midst of a challenging conversation, or while waiting for a meeting to begin. Allowing you to choose from the area currently requiring the most attention, the mindful breaks are organized around the three basic needs for thriving today: *Breathe* practices promote awareness, calm, and energy. *Becoming* practices offer us permission to fully be ourselves while addressing limiting beliefs, assertiveness, and confidence on the way to our goals and continued growth. *Balance* techniques focus on our values, priorities, and sustainable, ongoing recalibration.

Throughout you'll hear my personal experiences, reaffirming the effectiveness of these mindful breaks for everyday use. The mindful breaks enable us to not just live a mindful life but also enjoy more mindfulness in service of our own wellbeing as women and the realization of our most deeply held values.

I wrote *Don't Forget to Breathe* to offer support, wisdom, encouragement, and solutions for the busyness struggle we all face. I wrote it as a reminder to you and to myself that mindfulness is about living a fuller, happier, more balanced life. I love my kids, I love my husband, my friends, my hobbies, and my work. With these many priorities I can become easily, barely perceptively lulled into a pattern of imbalance. I know how much better it feels and how much more effective I am when I have found a more mindful balance. Because, ultimately, when we are mindful is when the magic happens and when we achieve what matters most to each of us.

Actually, It's ALL about Balance

Aaaarrrrgghhhh, I exhaled forcefully through gritted teeth, emitting a sound similar to a disgruntled pirate. Immediately, I felt my jaw tense and blood pressure spike, caught off-guard by this uncharacteristic bit of *read rage*—that burst of reactive anger akin to road rage experienced while perusing a frustrating piece of writing.

I had just flopped down on the couch with my morning coffee and laptop, happily anticipating a leisurely scroll through emails, when, *before ingesting even one sip of my precious coffee*, I encountered a full-on rant about the utterly BS-filled impossibility of work–life balance. *Aaaggrrrhhh!*

Nearly every book geared toward women I've recently encountered contains a chapter on the feasibility of work–life balance. And though the discourse is once again having its moment in the spotlight, the debate is certainly not new. The wide-ranging topic of work–life balance has been around for the entirety of my career and, I'm sure, long before that. Though far from a paragon of infinite patience, it's rare that I succumb to read rage, especially at an early, uncaffeinated hour. This latest rant, however, left me thinking, *Here we go again.* I inhaled deeply and sighed.

I am TIRED of reading and hearing that balance is impossible, that balance is BS, that we need to forget about balance! And though I generally appreciate both a healthy debate and the importance of semantics, focusing on the argument itself diverts all our powerful female energy *away from* playing big and actually creating the balance we spend so much precious time debating.

Believe me, I get it. I understand it is a continual discussion because we so desperately want work–life balance to be both possible and true. We are all yearning for a similar outcome: happiness, engagement, enjoyment, a fulfilling life that is full yet *not too full.*

You are TIRED of the debate, yet here you are engaging in it?, you ask, perceptively. I know. For the most part, I am fairly proficient at choosing my battles. When I find myself grumbling like a pirate, however, it's likely *past time* for me to speak up.

Instead of work–life balance, I prefer to call it simply *life balance*, as this more globally encapsulates the varied, ever-evolving facets of our lives. Instead of debating whether work–life balance is possible, let's redirect all that passionate energy to the ongoing recalibration of overall balance in our lives.

First, we must address which definition of life balance is being applied. I call this the Land of Fairy Tales versus *Real Life* Balance. In the Land of Fairy Tales, the beautiful, career-driven princess sashays through her days, perpetual smile on her face, sing-songy voice without the slightest hint of stress, each piece of her blissful life playing out precisely as planned, all Instagram-worthy, sublimely effortless, and perfectly balanced.

Sure, we may occasionally *fantasize* about this, but who among us actually *believes* it? We've been around long enough to know there is no one-size-fits-all life balance prescription. We are fully, sometimes painfully, aware that the Real Life Balance ebbs and flows as life happens, whether by choice, circumstance, or stage of life. If the Land of Fairy Tales is your working definition of balance, then agreed, it is an unattainable boatload of BS.

You may be wondering, *What, then, is a healthy life balance?* It's a gentle, ongoing recalibration of priorities through the ever-evolving seasons of life. In this book, I invite you to playfully experiment.

Life balance involves regularly adjusting your time and energy, making deliberate choices, lessening the guilt, (dare I say) lowering expectations, and accepting that you may not be able to have it all, or do it all, at once. Life balance is categorically imperfect and absolutely attainable.

This imperfect, dynamic balance formula is unique to each of us and changes continuously—sometimes due to a huge, life-altering event, or as the result of a much more subtle shift in our growth as a person. The good news is that it can actually be FUN. It's all about our perception, attitude, and definition and not at all about a perfect, all-or-nothing condition.

Despite our society's heralding of the busy employee and the false narrative of needing to be stressed out and overworked in order to be productive and serious about one's career, in reality, we also require play, self-care, and space in our schedules in order to function at our best. Because when even one aspect of our lives, either personal or professional, is out of balance, the resulting stress seeps into our thoughts, emotions, reactions, and behaviors in *all* facets of our lives. We run on autopilot—unintentional in our actions, repeating unhealthy habits. To avoid the anxious feelings, we binge on Ben & Jerry's, numb with mojitos, zone out with social media, or cultivate workaholic tendencies. And when we are depleted, we are not very productive or innovative and certainly not operating at our best.

At the end of a long week, when mental and physical energy reserves are at their lowest, there is scant opportunity for reflection or insight into improving our wearying plight. We spend the weekend recuperating and preparing for the busy onslaught to commence once again early Monday morning, perhaps even crawling out of bed in the wee hours of the morning to check our email.

Without regularly pausing to step back and survey the big picture, it is impossible to assess the ineffectiveness of our long-standing habits or how we might better prioritize. Not only that, but when we are stressed and slip into survival mode, the first things to go are the good stuff: our sense of humor, compassion, clarity of thought, and libido. We lose sight of what matters most deeply to us: connecting with family and friends, engaging in hobbies for the sake of pure enjoyment, offering ourselves a little well-deserved TLC. Instead, we fill our time with whatever appears urgent in the moment—typically *everything but* what matters most. We become so habitually conditioned to stress that we may not even recognize the tension headaches, achy muscles, or stomach ailments until our health deteriorates to the point of complete exhaustion, illness, or burnout—swiftly bringing us and our nonstop tendencies to an inevitable, screeching halt.

There's another way to live. We can pause, take a few deep breaths, and bring our full attention back to the present moment. This is the practice of mindfulness, which helps us slow the seemingly urgent pace of our lives. With mindfulness, we are better able to choose where we place our attention, determine our response rather than reacting habitually, notice and savor beautiful moments, and create increased calm. When we are calm, we are more creative, playful, efficient, healthy, and happy.

After I regained my composure, post-*read rage*, I started to wonder . . . what is *so appealing* about surrendering the possibility of life balance? What is it about completely giving up on the idea of balance that compels bright, ambitious women to put down their valuable work, pick up their phones, and launch into an impassioned, anti-balance rant?

And then it hit me. *Permission.* It's all about permission.

Permission *from ourselves* to ditch the damaging perfectionism. Permission to stop striving, grinding, hustling, nonstop to-do-listing. Permission to just, well, STOP.

I am all for it, and I completely get it. We've all been there: desperately craving the impossible luxury of hopping off the hamster wheel and disappearing for a few days. Yearning for rest, for time to regroup, recharge, to smell the roses and maybe, I don't know, *enjoy life*. Yes, yes, one hundred times yes.

Consider *Don't Forget to Breathe* your official permission slip to ditch damaging ideas of perfectionism—and, instead, take care of yourself. Self-care is essential—that is, knowing when to stop and how to rest, to calm our nervous systems, crawl under the covers with a good book, soak in the tub with a glass of wine, nourish ourselves with a warm bowl of comfort food.

Once we've rested, reset, and gotten our bearings, then what? More rest? More permission *not* to concern ourselves with creating a full, engaged, well-lived life? Umm, hell no.

Of course, there are times we simply want to breathe and care for ourselves. There are also times we want more—to hustle, grow, and push the boundaries. Periods of resting and those of striving. *It's all about the balance.*

What you'll find within these pages is the flexible framework to recalibrate in a way that works for you. *Don't Forget to Breathe* shares simple tools to increase our capacity for mindfulness, assertiveness, empowerment, and engagement, regardless of occupation. To be tuned in, at ease, and aware of our overarching goals is a powerful recipe for overall success. Only then can we tweak our life structure and choices in small ways, ushering overall balance into our daily lives. Let's get to it.

Real Talk for the Real World

I am keenly aware that many of the stressors discussed within this book may be deemed champagne, first-world problems. One might question, as I have, if it is hedonistic to focus so heavily on ourselves while there are serious world issues yet to be addressed. I cannot emphasize enough that when we are not whole, healthy, and balanced ourselves, we are not equipped with the energy, attention, or compassion necessary to care for anyone else. When weathering a rough patch in our lives—whether a loss, major change, or various stressors simultaneously—we become highly self-focused, which is a necessity at such times in order to cope, solve, and grow. There is no need to judge ourselves for the stressors or our reactions to them. Instead, we can use these simple mindfulness practices to slowly nudge ourselves in the direction of calm, balance, and health so we can once again be a positive force in the world, whatever form that takes. For it is during those times when life feels balanced and calm that we can look up and outward at the world and assess our part in creating a better one—whether through simple interactions with family, at work, or in the community at large. When we ourselves are whole, we have the capacity to care for others and to make our own unique, invaluable contributions for the greater good.

We've Come a Long Way, Baby— But Have We?

The challenge to all of us is to live a revolution,
not die for one.
—Gloria Steinem

"Mindfulness for *women*? What about men? Don't they need mindfulness, too?" I'm frequently asked this question, uttered exclusively by men. I understand the sentiment, I do, and categorically harbor no ill will against the male species (my loving father is one, I am happily married to one, and I am raising an adorable one). Obviously, men also struggle with stress and deserve to live calm, mindful lives. Absolutely, I want them to learn and benefit from mindfulness. The fact is, however, that although much progress has been made in the arena of male-female equality, we women still confront distinct obstacles specific to our gender—such as unequal representation, pay, and leadership opportunities in the workplace; society's unspoken but ubiquitous expectations of Superwoman; and a common dose of self-doubt—all while attempting to appear consistently polished and put together.

It is imperative that we raise and educate men to be aware, mindful, and compassionate. But until true gender equality has been reached, there is still a vital need to address women-specific issues. Franchesca Ramsey, writer, actress, and vlogger, wisely uses the analogy of taking part in a breast cancer race. Walking to raise funds for breast cancer research in no way suggests that pediatric cancer is not just as worthy a cause; it's simply that at that moment I am bringing awareness to the issue of breast cancer. Period. It need not be an either-or issue—mindfulness for women isn't one, either.

According to research, women are nearly twice as likely as men to suffer from severe anxiety and stress.[1] We women are desperate to simplify and streamline our lives yet are perplexed as to where exactly in the overflowing schedule doing so fits or how to even begin. Despite the popularity of mindfulness in modern society, we appear to be moving further and further away from actually living mindful lives. It seems the more we attempt to simplify and get quiet, the louder the societal forces shout at us that busy equals productive. We are not only working outside the home but routinely managing it as well. Constant organizing, planning, remembering, and toggling between countless work–life details is a baffling combination, bound to distract and overwhelm. This, my friend, is why I've created the quick but powerful mindful breaks—so we can reset and refocus while getting it all done *mindfully*.

In *Drop the Ball*, Tiffany Dufu writes about the myth of the ideally supported worker, in which, à la outdated *Mad Men* or *Leave It to Beaver*, "The professional world assumes that every full-time employee has someone else managing his or her home." When, in reality, according to McKinsey and Company's 2017 Women in the Workplace study, "women with a partner and children are 5.5

times more likely than their male counterparts to do all or most of the household work. And even when women are primary bread-winners, they do more work at home. Women who bring in more than fifty percent of their family income are 3.5 times more likely to do all or most of the household work than men in the same situation."[2] Overwhelming and exhausting, oh yes. This is precisely where the powerful Breathe Mindful Breaks come to the rescue.

We are navigating these everyday life stressors and also facing the more subtle, insidious gender–workplace inequities. Due to the sense of scarcity for leadership opportunity within a primarily male professional environment, for example, typically affable, collaborative women can become unfavorably competitive with one another. It needn't be this way. To counteract this natural instinct, we can be attentive to its arising, offer ourselves compassion for the struggle, then purposefully connect, support, and promote one another's interests in the workplace. While genuinely seeking to understand and respect rather than judge each other, we model, teach, and lift each other up with encouragement. In order to come together in this collaborative, unified manner, though, we must each first feel strong and confident in ourselves and our abilities. To help you build these skills see the mindful breaks in chapter 2. When in need of a shot of confidence or assertiveness, the Becoming Mindful Breaks are just what the doctor ordered.

Furthermore, in a male-dominated work world, the rest of us may find it challenging to communicate in a genuine and sensitive manner, sensing the need to be "on" all the time, fearful of exhibiting any vulnerability, lest it be held or used against us. With mindfulness practice, however, it is easier to observe self-doubt, self-criticism, and the subconscious stifling of personality that can originate from concern about being disliked or not taken seriously. Only when we recognize the existing barriers can we adjust our behavior so it is not driven by fear or negativity but rather by deliberate, authentic action. Recognizing when to alter our speed, edit our priorities, and redesign our goals are exactly the practical steps found within the Balance Mindful Breaks.

Through my years of balance work with women—moms with busy teens, leaders in the business world, artists honing their crafts—I have come to appreciate that we all share similar struggles regardless of life phase or occupation. And lest I have painted a demoralizingly bleak picture of the female landscape, I want you to know that I have great hope for us all. Conditions are slowly improving.

Change *is* happening. But it is also up to us. It begins with each one of us individually doing what we can to rebalance—which is precisely why I have written *Don't Forget to Breathe*. For you. For myself. So we women can recognize what we need to heal in order to become whole, strong, and steady. I see bright, wise, fearless women of all ages all around. By evoking the best in ourselves we can uncover the best in each other. We all benefit from mindful awareness, learning to be authentic, reaching for success, and uncovering the power to create balance. Whether we are managing a corporation or a household, mindfulness teaches us how to be the best possible version of ourselves, benefiting our families, our workplace, and the world—both men and women.

Caring for myself is not self-indulgence, it is self-preservation, and that is an act of political warfare.

—Audre Lorde

Mindfulness: What's All the Hype?

Almost everything will work again if you unplug it for a few minutes, including you.

—Anne Lamott

We've all had that experience of hopping in our car and driving to a familiar destination only to realize that we have very little recollection of making a specific turn or passing a well-known landmark. Operating on automatic pilot, we were not fully aware of our surroundings, which begs the question, Where in the world *were* we? Well, our thoughts were either in the future (worrying, what-iffing, mentally running through the to-do list) or in the past (rehashing a recent conversation or a long-ago memory) but certainly not inhabiting the present moment. Research by Matthew Killingsworth shows that our busy minds wander nearly half of our waking hours![3] Mindfulness, the direct opposite of automatic pilot, is intentionally bringing our awareness to what is happening in the moment, with the added attitude of kindness and acceptance.

Another way to conceptualize mindfulness is with the Triangle of Awareness. Imagine a triangle, the three points corresponding to our body sensations, thoughts, and emotions. These three points are very much interconnected and impact one another rapidly, often without our knowledge. Let's look at an example to illustrate this.

Jane, a marketing coordinator at a large hospital, relishes the various interactive, dynamic aspects of her position. She loves the variety of tasks, the flexibility of her schedule, and the perfect mix of solo and collaborative projects. Her supervisor, Susan, however, is not always so lovable. Though Susan can be generous and affable, she can also, in the blink of an eye, turn angry, impulsive, and mean-spirited. It is this disconcerting unpredictability that Jane finds most nerve-racking. Having worked with Susan long enough (three years, seven months, and twenty-three days, but who's counting?), Jane knows full well that the intense outburst will at least be happily short lived. Before long, Susan will predictably return to "normal," though not without leaving a trail of anxiety, bruised egos, and mounting resentments in her wake.

One early morning as Jane was contentedly preparing for a high-powered focus group later that day, Susan stormed into her office, red-faced, spitting anger-infused words through gritted teeth. "Tara sent out the document with a massive error! We cannot have this! It reflects horribly on all of us! What a disaster!"

Freeze. What is happening right now in Jane's Triangle of Awareness? Her thoughts: *Oh no, what's happened?!* Body sensations: heart racing, muscle tension, and the catching of breath in her throat. Emotions: utter surprise and confusion. Jane's next thoughts: *What if I lose my job? How will I pay my bills?* Body sensations: tight chest, raised shoulders, and heat rising up her face. Emotions: fear and panic.

As Jane continues spinning wretchedly around the triangle in an emotionally charged loop, a cascade of reactions in the form of fight-or-flight also begins to take shape. Fight-or-flight is our body's automatic reaction to perceived danger, quite adaptive and helpful when faced with a true threat. If, for instance, you are strolling across a busy street and glance up to see a car barreling toward you at high speed, your fight-or-flight response kicks in: adrenaline flows and your heart quickly pumps blood to your muscles, enabling you to efficiently leap out of harm's way.

Fight-or-flight affects activity in the brain as well. The front part of the brain, called the prefrontal cortex (responsible for attention, organization, and the capacity to step back and see the big picture), slows down its functioning, whereas the amygdala (in charge of emotional reactivity) fires rapidly, maintaining the ability to negotiate the threat. The dilemma is that in our busy lives, we perceive danger *all over the place* when in actuality there is none.

Although Jane is essentially safe in her office, her mind and body do not distinguish between a true threat and mere perceived danger, and thus fight-or-flight is swiftly engaged. Depending on her level of mindfulness in the moment, Jane's scenario could play out in one of two ways: If she is not on her mindful game that morning, she might become emotionally hijacked, her anger matching that of Susan's. Together, they'd continue the useless rant, wasting precious time and energy better spent on a workable solution.

If, however, Jane is able to recognize her raised shoulders and tight chest, she is cued in to the need for a few slow, deep breaths—in, out, in, out—thereby alerting her brain to the false alarm. Fight-or-flight decelerates, allowing the front part of her brain to once again operate efficiently. No longer emotionally hijacked but instead aware of her Triangle, Jane is able to *choose* her response rather than react out of anxiety and fear. By calming her fight-or-flight reaction, she is now in control, able to see clearly this all-too-familiar Susan cycle playing itself out. Jane, carefully maintaining her equilibrium in spite of Susan's spinning out of control, lets Susan know she will handle it, and while walking down the hall to Tara's office she continues to breathe deeply. By the time she reaches Tara's door, Jane is able to reasonably discuss the mishap, brainstorm solutions, and remedy the error. One might only imagine the alternative, unmindfully played-out scenario. By bringing our attention to any of the three points on the Triangle of Awareness, we are more able to manage our reactions to frustrating situations—from bumper-to-bumper traffic to paralyzing to-do lists to those maddening, intractable colleagues.

Though the origins of mindfulness can be traced to Buddhism, it is a completely secular way of training the mind and brain, albeit a powerful adjunct to religious affiliation and prayer. And despite its ubiquitous appearance in the mainstream media, it is not simply a passing fad. Mindfulness is an evidence-based practice supported by a huge body of research, which is why countless organizations such as Google, Aetna, General Mills, Intel, Goldman Sachs, and Dow Chemical Company offer employee training in mindfulness. Research indicates that regular mindfulness practice leads to a decrease in employee sick time and reported stress levels; an increase in overall sense of well-being, creativity, innovation, and collaboration; and a more positive work environment with happier, more engaged employees. In addition, a study focused on mindful communication with family physicians indicates less burnout and stress, with an increase in resilience and overall mood.[4] Research shows that mindfulness not only reduces stress but also trains the capacity of mind not often receiving attention and thus has been referred to as a "superpower." With studies by the hundreds it is clear that mindfulness is good for employees, leaders, organizations, and the health and well-being of all.

Meditation: It's Not What You Think

I think ninety-nine times and I find nothing. I stop thinking,
swim in the silence, and the truth comes to me.
—Albert Einstein

I am not a huge fan of spectator sports. My six-year-old, however, has recently developed a love affair with all things basketball, including our hometown favorite, the Philadelphia 76ers. The other day as I sat with my husband and son to watch a few minutes of a game, the discussion turned to star player Ben Simmons. As my guys chatted about Simmons's skill, focus, and aptitude for teamwork, I observed him gracefully traveling down the court with full attention. "I'll bet he meditates," I instinctively, confidently professed. My husband chuckled at what he supposed was an offhand remark, but I was serious. Simmons exudes that calm, focused attention arising from long-term meditation. So, reacting as any respectable person compelled to be proved right would, I darted to my laptop and googled, "Does Ben Simmons meditate?" Apparently, my mindfulness radar is in good working order—Ben Simmons has practiced meditation as part of his athletic mental skills training *since he was eleven years old. Bam!*

I spent a few brief moments smugly relishing my intuitive genius, though in retrospect I loathsomely admit it wasn't such an extraordinary realization. From years of reading about and teaching mindfulness, I am privy to the knowledge that the team members of the Chicago Bulls, Seattle Seahawks, San Francisco 49ers, Atlanta Falcons and many athletes in various sports all now meditate. But, in my fleeting, yet pompously swaggering defense, none of this was at the forefront of my mind as I merely watched a young man command a basketball game with a seemingly unflappable, focused sense of ease. *Bam* again.

Of course we are all unique in our innate level of calm and emotional reactivity. In all fairness, perhaps as a child Ben was as chill as they come. Some of us remain seemingly unfazed by relentless chaos while others react dramatically at the slightest deviation from calm. Regardless, the good news is that we can train ourselves to be more mindful and nonreactive despite our natural disposition, age, or life circumstance. And, thankfully, we need not be professionally trained athletes or eleven years old in order to garner the far-reaching benefits of mindfulness meditation. With regular practice, these mindfulness skills are translatable to any area of our lives, in any situation, with any goal or dream; because when we are calm, focused, and at ease, we are more able to function at peak ability.

If mindfulness is intentionally paying attention to the present moment with a nonjudgmental attitude in the midst of any daily activity, what exactly, then, is meditation? Meditation is *carving out uninterrupted time to practice the skill of mindfulness.* When we meditate, we choose a point of focus (for example, the natural rising and falling of the belly as the breath comes and goes), observe when our attention wanders off (which it does for everyone countless times), and repeatedly and kindly return our attention to the chosen point of focus (the home base of the breath).

Habits do not restrict freedom. They create it.

—James Clear

It is wholly unnecessary to twist oneself into a pretzel, chant om, or burn incense in order to do this. Sitting comfortably in a chair or on a cushion on the floor works just fine. It is necessary, however, to practice regularly. Just as if you were learning to play piano or basketball, it's not possible to simply read about it or attempt it one time and expect to play like Beethoven or Ben Simmons. The same goes for meditation. We need to do it regularly to build our mindfulness skill of attention. A daily meditation practice lays the foundation for a life of more calmness, ease, and overall mindfulness.

Meditation is *not* (I repeat, *not*) about clearing our mind of thoughts (sorry about the shouty italics, but I need to hit this one home, as it is by far the most common misconception I encounter). Our minds are *designed* to think thoughts. Instead, meditation is about familiarizing ourselves with our incessant thoughts and allowing them to settle. A snow globe is a great analogy. When we are stressed and overwhelmed, our minds are like the snow globe after it is vigorously shaken—rendering it impossible to see clearly through the scattered flakes. When we take a few deep breaths, our thoughts and bodies calm a bit, the snow globe equivalent of the flakes settling to the bottom. The stressors have not disappeared, but we now have a clearer perspective, allowing for more creative thought, enhanced problem solving, and reconnecting with what most matters as the unimportant falls away. If this is the power of a few mindful breaths, imagine the benefits of five full minutes of meditation.

Amazingly, research now shows that ongoing meditation practice literally changes the shape and function of the brain. The prefrontal cortex (the part of the brain responsible for problem solving, planning, and emotion regulation) and the hippocampus (responsible for memory and learning) physically increase in size while the amygdala (connected to fight-or flight and emotional reactivity) decreases in size with regular meditation practice.[5] Not only that, but connections between certain areas of the brain are weakened while others are strengthened, resulting in less emotional reactivity and increased capacity for concentration and attention.

Our world is often one of constant chatter unless we deliberately seek out a bit of silence. For some, the thought of silence strikes terror in their hearts while for others it is a welcome respite from sensory overload. For many it has been a really long time since encountering a significant period of quiet. Much of this depends on whether we are an introvert or extrovert, our stage in life, and how much sensory stimulation we encounter on a regular basis. Without creating time for silence, for space in our lives, we deprive ourselves and others of our capacity to be the best we can be as friends, partners, moms, employees, and women. What I have found from teaching meditation is that once we have tasted silence, we begin to crave it. Sitting quietly and noticing thoughts without being pulled into the emotion of them enables insight and clarity as a positive guiding force in our lives.

Let's Do It!

When: You may need to experiment with various times of day to meditate to find the time that suits you best. When you hit upon one, stick with it. Routines are most easily formed if we bookend them between two already established habits; for example, waking in the morning, washing your face, sitting to meditate, and then enjoying your cup of coffee. I have found that early morning is the ideal time for me, while my house is still quiet. I also love how it sets the tone for my day. You may prefer winding down at bedtime, behind your closed office door at lunchtime, or transitioning after returning home from work. Your meditation time might also vary depending on your changing daily agenda. Regardless, ink it into your schedule as one of your top priorities.

Where: As best you can, find a quiet place where you will not be disturbed. Set firm boundaries with yourself, your family, your pets, and if applicable, your staff, that you should be interrupted only in case of emergency. Of course, we cannot control all variables; we may hear outside traffic or a conversation in the hallway. Simply allow these sounds to become part of your meditation. If you are able to find a spot outdoors where you will not be disturbed, this can also be a lovely way to meditate.

Why (am I doing this again?): Inevitably there will come a time when you wonder why in the world you are sitting for five entire minutes presumably accomplishing nothing. Simply recognize this as doubt and to be expected. Remind yourself that you are taking this time to exercise your mind and brain. Much like you would do squats to strengthen your glutes, each time you redirect your attention to the home base of focus, you build that mindfulness muscle of attention (butt exercises for your brain?). Once you have established a regular meditation habit, you will miss it when you don't practice and will look forward to this time to nurture yourself. Give yourself time to get there.

How: It's helpful to begin with a guided audio recording. You can visit my website shondamoralis.net to download a free five-minute guided meditation (and coffee meditation!) or use one of the many apps now available (see Resource Guide, page 277). As it becomes increasingly familiar and comfortable, you may find you prefer practicing on your own and lengthening the amount of meditation time.

To begin meditating, first find a chair in which your feet comfortably touch the ground, or sit on the floor atop pillows so your bottom and hips are raised. Sit up tall, straighten the spine, relax the shoulders, and allow the eyes to close. With a sense of curiosity, notice the various body sensations. Slowly scan through each part, beginning with the feet and systematically moving up to the head. Notice any areas of tightness. Are your shoulders raised toward your ears? Is your brow furrowed? Can you soften those areas and relax the small muscles around your eyes and mouth?

Now relax your belly, noticing how it rises and falls as the breath comes and goes. There is no need to take deeper breaths or change it in any way. See if you can notice the beginning and ending of the inhale, the beginning and ending of the exhale, and, perhaps, a pause happening naturally in between. When your attention wanders off the breath, silently note where it was—planning, remembering, judging, imagining, thinking—then gently return your attention to the breath in the belly and begin again. You may judge the drifting off with thoughts like, *What is wrong with you? Why can't you stay focused on the breath for longer than twenty seconds?!* Silently note this as "judging," and come back to the breath. Each time your mind wanders, kindly bring it back to the sensations of breathing in the belly. If your mind wanders off fifty times within your five minutes, you return to the breath at fifty-one.

How Long: Start with an achievable five minutes a day. Reactions to this suggestion vary almost comically, ranging anywhere from *Only five?* to *You want me to sit still for five whole minutes?* And then there is the type A, overly ambitious response, *If five minutes is good, forty-five must* *be even better! I think I'll do that!* I encourage all of you, regardless of your gut reaction, to begin with five. If five minutes feels excruciatingly long, one minute is perfectly fine. It is much more critical that we establish a *daily* meditation habit than concern ourselves with the length of it. When we keep it short, simple, and manageable, we eventually want to sit a bit longer. For now, enjoy those five minutes each day, gradually crafting a lifelong habit of meditation and mindfulness.

Let go of expectations and observe what arises. The goal of meditation itself is not relaxation, though it is often a welcome side effect. Paying attention may require some effort, but we must take care to avoid trying too hard, relax our attitude, and focus. Bring an attitude of curiosity and playfulness to your meditation time. Consistency and flexibility are also essential. Oh yes, and a healthy sense of humor. The multitude of random thoughts that show up can be quite amusing.

Each time you meditate, congratulate yourself for carving out the time, sitting, and staying put. Cultivate this attitude of awareness outside of your meditation time with a handful of mindful breaks. Really, what good is your meditation if you immediately commence dashing frantically through the next part of your day? That, my friend, is precisely what the mindful breaks are meant to ward against.

How to Use the Breathe, Becoming, and Balance Mindful Breaks

The secret of getting ahead is getting started.
—Agatha Christie

It's easy to lament the number of ways that our lives are not working the way we'd like: too many responsibilities, not enough time, overall life imbalance, and resulting guilt. It is not so easy to envision and put into practice exactly how we *would* like our day-to-day lives to play out. We attempt to change too many pieces at once, experience all sorts of resistance, become inundated and grow weary, and surrender to those long-standing, familiar, yet unhelpful, routines. Motivation screeches to a sudden halt and back to square one we go (with our inner critic heaping on a hearty dose of guilt along the way).

Though we are not always in control of what life throws our way, we are the authors of our own lives, and how we cope is completely up to us. This book is designed to encourage us to address our mental limitations and grow beyond them; to be productive and happy without fixating on daily stressors; to reach our personal and professional goals; and to find balance in our lives by recognizing how and when to recalibrate.

The 5-minute mindful breaks do not require extra time; only that you bring your full attention to a part of your day that is *already happening*—and *actually be aware* that it is happening. You will find that these breaks help you experience more energy, efficiency, productivity, and calmness. Eventually, by investing in those few minutes throughout the day, you will gain more time overall.

There are three types of mindful breaks in this book: *Breathe* practices help us become more calm and aware. *Becoming* breaks promote growth, goals, and confidence. And the *Balance* breaks help us recalibrate and achieve success. Each builds upon and supports the other in what I call the *Don't Forget to Breathe Upward Spiral*. We pull out and use certain mindful breaks depending on what is called for in the moment or in our particular season of life.

The upward spiral framework helps us thrive, adapt, and recalibrate balance for the rest of our lives. The upward spiral is an invitation—an exciting, ongoing, lifelong trajectory of growth using self-awareness and calm to unleash our superpowers in a way that is mindful and sustainable.

If that level of excitement makes you feel like curling up on the couch under a blanket and taking a nap, that's perfectly fine (and I've got a mindful break for that). Though we do want to live rich, full lives, we also don't want to be pushing and striving all the time. That would not be the most balanced way to live.

There are times when we will need to coast for a while, rest, allow all that juicy creativity to ferment, take in the view, and perhaps care for others or ourselves in earnest. These are opportunities to practice deep self-compassion, allowing life to unfold as it will and observing it mindfully. This is where the Breathe mindful breaks come in handy.

After we are reasonably rested and calm, we might want to stretch ourselves and embark on a new habit or endeavor. It is in these times of stepping out of our comfort zone, when we are on the verge of a breakthrough, right on the cusp of growth, when those pesky limiting beliefs show up. You know: *Who am I? I'm not ready. I'm not [fill in the blank] enough.* These are precisely the times that call for a shot of assertiveness, bravery, and those confidence-boosting Becoming breaks.

And then, in some moments and seasons of life, we feel compelled to follow our curiosity and play bigger. Though exciting, it can also feel overwhelming and paralysis-inducing. This is when we pull out those Balance breaks to help us clarify our dreams, stay true to our values, and create those specific, attainable goals. On the way to those dreams, we benefit from pausing to assess the speed, fullness, and level of energy expenditure. The Balance mindful breaks help us recalibrate our overall life balance in an ongoing and adaptable yet sustainable way. By noticing when the balance has skewed toward too busy or too stagnant, we pull out an appropriate Balance mindful break for the occasion, then coax ourselves kindly but firmly back into a relative state of equilibrium. And off we go.

Here's how to do it:

❶ One break at a time. Rather than overwhelm our-selves with many transformations at once, we can delib-erately create the best conditions within our control *with one tiny action-step at a time,* each contributing to a positive, far-reaching ripple effect. Those tiny action-steps compose many of the mindful breaks. Like a single droplet of water released onto the still surface of a lake, one seemingly inconsequential change has a more wide-spread positive impact on our lives than we might ever imagine at first glance.

❷ Which break is calling your name? There are dozens of mindful breaks, so flip to a page that resonates with you in any particular moment. (Or by all means read the book cover to cover and then choose.) The breaks are fun exper-iments, achievable challenges, and quick calming tricks to keep in your back pocket for when you need them most. Whichever breaks you choose, keep them simple and fun. Start with one and see where it takes you.

- The **Breathe Mindful Breaks** promote calm and aware-ness. They are tools to help you find peace in any situation.

- The **Becoming Mindful Breaks** enable you to notice and modify limiting self-beliefs, power up assertiveness skills, increase and sustain energy, and bolster self-confidence.

- The **Balance Mindful Breaks** coach you to stay true to your values, keep priorities in check, and maintain relative equilibrium through the ever-evolving seasons of life.

❸ **Change 'em up and make them work for you.** There is no one-size-fits-all mindful break. I encourage you to modify them to suit your needs. They appeal to a continuum of personality traits. For example, some of us are more natural risk takers while others prefer to play it safe; some love to exercise while others find the idea abhorrent. Practicing the mindful breaks from your own unique starting point will yield the best results.

❹ **Layer the breaks incrementally.** Slowly, over time, pepper your days with mindful breaks as you add one or two to your repertoire each week. Before long you will be amazed at how tiny adjustments can create far-reaching transformations in your life.

❺ **Then change 'em up again.** Investigating where we fall on each continuum of personality traits offers a more informed place to start and can (and should) be recalibrated when necessary. As our overall self-awareness is heightened, we can more intricately adapt each break to fit our own unique, ever-changing needs while continuing to identify which other mindful breaks can be integrated into our lives.

❻ **Meditation + mindful breaks = your ultimate mindful edge.** Try meditating for five minutes each day in addition to sprinkling mindful breaks throughout, for it is the *combination of the two* that packs the most powerful one-two punch. Daily meditation lays the groundwork for overall mindful awareness, and the breaks enable you to weave more mindfulness throughout your days.

❼ Keep it short to start. If you find that 5-minute mindful breaks are too long, begin with one minute, which is one minute more than you were practicing previously. Once you taste a bit of mindfulness, you will soon be searching for opportunities to add more of it to your day.

❽ Keep it conspicuous. Leave *Don't Forget to Breathe* visible on your desk, on your living room coffee table, or on your bedroom nightstand as a reminder to pause and take a mindful break. What one small step will you take toward balance? Now take a deep breath and go get 'em.

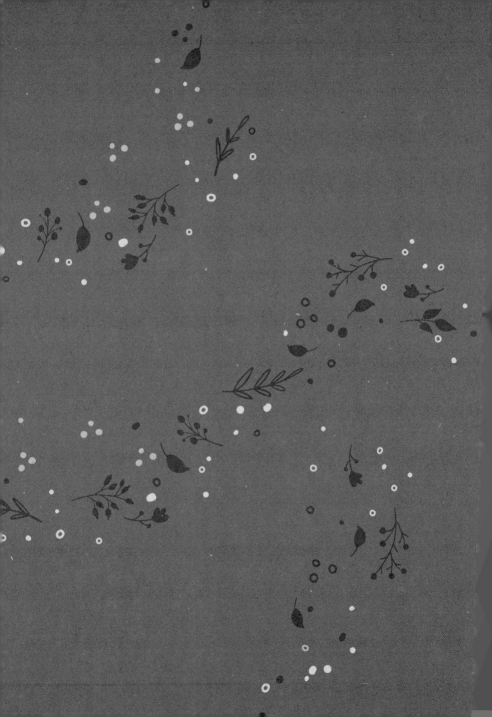

CHAPTER 1

Breathe Mindful Breaks

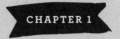

As busy women, we are often focused on checking items off the to-do list. Caught up in the buzz of doing, we can easily lose sight of our true priorities and thoughtful judgment. This hamster-wheel pace, naturally lending itself to shallow breathing in the chest, tense muscles, and an underlying sense of the scarcity of time and energy, is hardly the optimal state from which to operate. Aware of the unsustainable pace, we either mistakenly believe there is no other way to exist or are categorically overwhelmed with how to change the status quo. After all, when it seems as if there is not even enough time to *breathe fully*, how in the world do we find the time to map out another, better way to live?

This is exactly where Breathe Mindful Breaks come to the rescue. Both soothing and strategic, they are designed to bring us a bit of peace in any situation so that we can act and achieve with intentionality and purpose. Loosely ordered as to how they might unfold throughout the course of a day, they are brief moments of respite and calm, reminders that we have the capacity not only to survive but to thrive as well. Breathe Mindful Breaks pull us out of the constant swirling of thoughts and open up the space for wiser, more deliberate and creative reasoning. They are the grounding lifelines necessary for us to get things done while sustaining energy and clarity of mind. The Breathe Mindful Breaks are the answer you've been looking for—a different, more peaceful, engaged way to live. Go ahead, dive in. You will be amazed at just how powerful these short, accessible mindful breaks can be.

Coffee

—

Drink your tea slowly and reverently, as if it is the axis on which the world earth revolves—slowly, evenly, without rushing toward the future. Live the actual moment. Only this moment is life. **—Thich Nhat Hanh**

When I began meditating first thing in the morning well over a decade ago, I was intent on staying true to my daily half-hour session untouched by caffeine, social media, or human conversation. After rousing to my predawn alarm, I would shuffle to the bathroom, splash some shockingly cold (but oddly pleasant) water on my face, and soon be fairly awake and alert. On the occasional sleepy morning the fantasy of some pre-meditation coffee would arise, but I never actually indulged. The rule follower in me would have surely chastised loudly: *What would the great meditation teachers think of that? Tsk-tsk.* So regardless of my level of sleepiness, the fullness of the schedule, or how early my workday was to begin, I sat for thirty uncaffeinated minutes, making a beeline straight to my beloved coffee maker as soon as that half hour was up. Confession time: My morning meditation has changed somewhat since that time. My older—questionably wiser—self has taken to breaking this rule on occasion, often with a hint of rebellion. I broke the rule initially by necessity as a result of inevitable real-life time constraints and the occasional sleepless night, but now I do it purely because I enjoy the habit. Yes, I often meditate while savoring my cup of coffee. I love the stuff. It may have saved my life on numerous occasions. In my estimation, it certainly deserves a meditation dedicated solely to its lovely qualities.

Whether you're a java aficionado like me or a tea lover, you can practice the Coffee Mindful Break with your caffeinated or decaffeinated beverage of choice.

The Coffee Mindful Break

A note of caution: Before you settle in and sit down in a haze of sleepy fog, take note of where you place your cup so as not to spill its contents all over the floor when you complete the mindful break. Trust me on this one.

Sit tall in a comfortable position, either in a chair or on a cushion on the floor. Holding your cup in both hands, feel the warmth radiating into your hands, feel the smooth or coarse texture of the mug. Slowly lift the mug to your nose and inhale the scent as if for the first time. Without judgment, notice what thoughts arise. Notice how the muscles in your arms know just what to do as they lift the cup to your mouth.

Despite the urge to ingest the caffeine as soon as humanly possible (sounds a little desperate, but I've been there), see if you can pause for a moment and observe what happens. Is your mouth watering in sweet anticipation? Are your thoughts screaming for you to *please take a giant swig already*? Just notice. Then, with deliberate action, place the cup to your lips. Now take that first glorious sip and hold the flavorful liquid in your mouth, tasting as fully as you can. As you swallow, experience the warmth moving its way down your throat and into your stomach. Pause. Take a breath before your next sip. As you do, notice what occurs in the body. Has your heart rate increased? Does your mind feel more alert? Are the sensations pleasant or unpleasant? Tuning into our body sensations offers us subtle information we might otherwise miss. Perhaps you relish the mental sharpness that occurs. Perhaps you realize the caffeine causes slight feelings of anxiety and you decide to live without. These sensations and reactions may also shift over time. Keep watching. Stay curious. Enjoy.

The Commute

Many times, the means are the ends. How we choose to act changes who we choose to become. The way we choose to get to where we're going defines what it's going to be like when we get there. **—Seth Godin**

Cars and buses and trains, oh my! Bluetooth and podcasts and Audible, oh . . . my . . . So many choices; infinite potential distractions. Depending on the length of our commute and how often we travel, we could be talking hours upon hours of our lives. Even if the commute is a breezy seven minutes like mine, this is time that can be spent wisely, which is why I invite us all to start out with a bit of mindful silence. Doing so allows us to bring awareness to the moment and thoughts to settle, ushering some intentionality into the remainder of our commute.

The days when I'm attempting to squeeze in as much as humanly possible are those when I hop in my car, turn on the news, and—if not met with immediately fascinating content—impatiently switch stations every eleven seconds. I'm driven by a sort of hyper-restlessness, eager for a feel-good dopamine hit in the form of an intriguing interview snippet or piece of breaking news.

Fortunately, because of loads of practice, I'm able to catch myself early on. I turn off the radio, resist the strong urge to switch it right back on (lest I miss something compelling), breathe deeply, and settle into the silence. When we purposefully pause in this way, we recognize the restlessness-driven desire for something, *anything,* to fill the void, and we also train ourselves to notice and savor the sunrise, the scenery, the silence. We reconnect with the knowledge that our body is attached to our frantically thought-churning head and can then relax tight muscles. We remind our bodies that there is indeed no emergency, that a fight-or-flight reaction is not currently required. Then, and only then, are we able to question the viability and helpfulness of old commuting habits and intentionally decide where we will place our precious attention and energy. Rather than operating in that unconscious, barely aware state of autopilot, we can arrive at work awake, refreshed, and ready to take on the day.

The Commute Mindful Break

❶ Ideally at the outset, designate at least a portion of your commute to silence. This could feel downright painful at first. You may experience an impossibly strong pull to fill up that silence with some music, a podcast, or perhaps, in a moment of full-on desperation, a back-and-forth conversation with yourself. The pull is to be expected; the break becomes easier with practice. Most people find the silence surprisingly refreshing after resisting those first few urges. Feel free to stretch out the quiet for as long as you'd like.

❷ End the period of silence with an intention for the day, in whatever form resonates with you, such as: *May I be patient. May I listen with an open mind. Remember to breathe deeply throughout the day. Have fun. Let the negativity roll off.*

❸ After you have pulled yourself out of automatic pilot with the quiet, you are free to spend the remainder of your commute however you would like. Play some well-chosen music, a podcast, a news update, or an audiobook.

❹ Check in every so often to assess the impact of your choice. Are you engaged, calm, at ease? Has the restlessness crept back in? Adjust accordingly.

❺ When you arrive at your destination, take note of how you feel—your amount of energy, sense of happiness, and level of mindfulness. Go ahead and offer yourself a high five.

❻ On the way home: Follow the steps above. This is also a great opportunity to transition from work to home, reflecting on how you want to walk through that front door, ideally feeling a bit of freshness, shaking off any negativity from the day. Add a sprinkle of gratitude for the end of the work day, your home, and your family.

Triangle Tune-In

If we hope to go anywhere or develop ourselves in any way, we can only step from where we are standing. If we don't really know where we are standing . . . we may only go in circles.
—Jon Kabat-Zinn

Lisa, a thirty-six-year-old high school English teacher in an unpredictably turbulent inner-city high school came to me for mindfulness coaching to help her cope with overwhelm, difficulty focusing, and irritability. There was a time, Lisa wistfully recalled, when she loved her job, thrived amid the variability, and awoke with anticipated enthusiasm for a classroom filled with swirling teenage hormones and energy. But now her workday was a constant chaotic flurry of overstimulation and fire extinguishing, and at home she was struggling to find any semblance of peace coping with her two young children's endless liveliness and constant motion.

A scarcity of her own energy, time, and patience caused unrelenting tension that spilled over into Lisa's interactions with her students and family. "I can't shut my mind off. It runs nonstop," she lamented. Lisa felt this most acutely upon climbing into bed each night exhausted, when, for the first time all day, her body was permitted to cease its constant motion. Feeling like she was barely keeping her head above water, she was also at a loss as to what to do about it. Shoulders slumped and eyes filling with tears, she told me that the thought of adding even one more small obligation—even if it would rescue her from being pulled under—seemed daunting and paralyzing. I knew exactly which mindful break would provide her with a lifeline to prevent her from drowning and pull her back to thriving.

We discussed her prevailing hamster-wheel lifestyle, emphasizing that mindful breaks do not necessarily require any additional time or energy, only pausing to shift our perspective in the moment. She was up for trying just about anything and agreed to give the Triangle Tune-In Mindful Break a go.

Lisa designated three times in her day when she would practice the Triangle Tune-In: first thing in the morning as she sat at her desk, prior to checking e-mail and before the students began trickling in; at the start of her lunch period, before she began mindlessly eating her sandwich; and after her students left for the day, once she had packed up and was ready to head home for the afternoon.

After two weeks, Lisa returned to my office, excited to share the positive changes she was experiencing. "The Triangle Tune-In catches me at just the right time—when my head is spinning, when I am feeling anxious about what's to come, when I am wondering how in the world I will get it all done. By stopping and taking a few deep breaths, I am reminded to relax my muscles. I can feel the calm wash over me. There is still so much to be done, but I can put things in perspective and reassure myself that everything will be OK."

By discovering a way to calm herself in the midst of a full, active life, Lisa's racing thoughts diminished and bedtime became much more peaceful. She was able to respond to her family and students with patience, and once again bring playfulness and fun into her life. Her ability to cope returned as well, with a noticeable sense of ease.

The three points on the Triangle of Awareness consist of our body sensations, thoughts, and emotions, each impacting the others intimately and rapidly. You can use the Triangle to bring you back to the present moment when you realize you have been running on automatic pilot, worrying about the future or rehashing the past. (See Mindfulness: What's All the Hype?, on page 17, for a more detailed example of the Triangle of Awareness as a helpful tool to conceptualize mindful awareness.)

Instead of reactively putting out fires and living in a fixed mindset of time and energy shortage, you can use this mindful break as a reminder to pause first and pull yourself out of the swirling, disorganized mess that is your mind in overwhelm. By resetting and refocusing, you can reacquaint yourself with the present in a more mindful way, with the kind admonishment to *be here now,* attending to one task at time.

The Triangle Tune-In Mindful Break

Pause, take a few deep breaths, and bring your full awareness to the three points on the Triangle of Awareness, in no particular order:

❶ Body sensations: Beginning with the feet, briefly scan upward through each body part, noticing sensations and releasing muscle tension in each area if you encounter it. It may be difficult to detect any sensation at first, but becomes easier with practice. For example, *I feel a dull ache in my forehead, over my eyes, and in my neck. My eyes burn and eyelids feel heavy. My legs, especially the calves, feel fatigued and heavy. Or, I feel light and full of energy. I notice my lips turned up in a smile and a feeling of warmth in my chest.*

❷ Thoughts: What are you thinking right now? Are you planning or imagining the future, distant or near? Are you evaluating how this is going? Do you wonder how in the world this mindfulness business can possibly work? Notice when you might be critiquing, avoiding, or clinging to thoughts. There is no need to judge ourselves for the judging. Instead, simply label the thoughts without getting pulled into the endless rabbit hole of why or how. For example, my thoughts are, *I can't really feel much in my body. What's wrong with me? I can't even do this right* (judging thought). Or, *Wow, I am hungry. Oh shoot, I still need to stop at the store for groceries on the way home* (planning). *Or,* I have to write that report for tomorrow's meeting. Stop! No thinking about work after work *(planning, thinking, judging).*

❸ Emotions: With a sense of curiosity and acceptance, observe which emotions are present. They may be neutral or subtle and, unless highly charged, are often the most challenging to identify. It is also common at first to mistake thoughts for emotions. For example, someone might say, "I wish I hadn't said that," is an emotion, but it is a thought. The emotion is likely guilt or sadness. Or, "I wanted to get out of there" (again, a thought with attendant emotions of fear, anxiety, or anger). Double-check that what you are identifying is indeed an emotion rather than a thought. Sometimes various conflicting emotions are swirling around at once. It is not unusual to feel love, gratitude, and sadness or anger, hurt, and jealousy simultaneously. There is no need to qualify or justify any of our emotions; they arise, we notice them and then accept them as best we can (whether we are a fan or not). At a later time, we choose how we want to respond to them.

The Triangle Tune-In can be used as a tool to reset when you find yourself spinning out in overwhelm (as was initially the case with Lisa) or more of a proactive method to maintain calm and focus throughout the day. Depending on circumstance and time allowed, experiment with a brief twenty-second Tune-In as well as a more leisurely two-minute break. Now that you are tuned back in to yourself and your Triangle, carry this awareness of the present moment into the next part of your day.

Desk Body Scan

Your body shapes your mind. Your mind shapes your behavior. And your behavior shapes your future.

—Amy Cuddy

Each of us has a signature pattern of holding stress in the body—there are certain muscles we tighten and common areas of tension. For some, anxiety manifests as fierce pressure, as if the head were stuck in a constricting vise; others bemoan a constant, aching discomfort in their neck and shoulders; while some suffer from stomach ailments that send them sprinting for the nearest restroom when worries abound. While we may be highly attuned to a few of our signature stress patterns, others may be more sporadic and inconspicuous, requiring some routine mindful sleuthing on our part.

Soon after I began practicing mindfulness it became clear to me that the region of my lower back and butt would tighten when I was feeling anxious or overwhelmed, resulting in muscle fatigue and soreness. One might surmise that my chronic stress would have graciously resulted in rock-hard glutes, but no, of course not.

The only notable secondary consequence was chronic sciatica, quite literally an irritating pain in my butt. How's that for irony?

There was no need to investigate this constellation of sensations closely, as the relentless, nagging discomfort made itself obvious. It was only after a few *years* of practice, though, that I began to notice how increased stress unconsciously caused me to tense my left calf muscle as well. One morning after an especially challenging confrontational couples therapy session, I recall wondering why in the world *only* my left calf was sore and fatigued. It took time and repetition to realize that this is one of my signature areas of stress. The past few years, I have morphed into more of a shoulder-and-neck-tension kinda girl, the tightness taking up residence after hours of working at a computer and reading. And so it goes.

You might ask: *Why in the world would I want to actually* focus *on areas of discomfort in my body?* Great question! Thanks for playing. Despite the prevalent, tempting tendency to disregard the intricate yet undeniable connection between our bodies and minds, it is vital to our overall physical and mental well-being that we pay closer attention. The purpose of the Desk Body Scan is threefold.

Number one is to pull us out of automatic pilot, bring us back to the present moment, and offer some immediate calm so that we are able to think clearly and prioritize wisely. Imagine how you might enter into the next meeting or conversation differently, perhaps more creatively, and with a more open-minded approach if given a moment to first pause and relax your body. (Even better, imagine if *all* your colleagues did the same.)

Two, the Desk Body Scan is a mindful break designed to bring your full awareness to the ever-changing body sensations in the middle of a busy day, teaching you to recognize which sensations are present in your body *in this moment*. Instead of walking around unaware that we have actual feeling, sensing *bodies* attached to our intellectual heads—bodies we tend to discount, minimize, or flat-out ignore—we become more intimately aware of our subtle physical sensations as well as how they change in nuance and in intensity. As with my own experience, your unique patterns can shift over time, so it is helpful to monitor them on an ongoing basis.

Finally, it is important to familiarize ourselves with common sensations and our signature stress areas because the more aware we are, the quicker we can cue in to when we are stressed, which, as in the case of my left calf muscle, is not always immediately apparent. Only when we are mindful are we able to act on our own behalf. Now when I notice an ache in my shoulders, it is a reminder to slowly drop them, take a deep breath, and sit up tall, perhaps adding a nice stretch, gently leaning my head back and gazing upward. It is also an opportunity for me to pause and inquire into my current overall level of stress, giving me valuable information to work with and the ability to make small, subtle recalibrations in my life.

The Desk Body Scan Mindful Break

You can practice this mindful break with eyes open or closed, depending on your level of privacy and comfort. Sit up tall. Imagine there is an invisible chord running from your tailbone, up through the spine, gently pulling skyward through the top of the head, elongating the back and neck. Drop your shoulders and allow your hands to rest on the armrests or your lap. Now bring your attention to the feet, noticing any subtle sensations such as warmth, coolness, or pressure where the shoes are touching the feet. With an attitude of curiosity, notice sensations in the ankles, lower legs, knees, and upper legs, allowing a few seconds to rest your awareness at each area. When thoughts arise (*Oh, that's right, I need shoes for my cousin's wedding! When will I get to the store? My pants are tight. I need to get back to the gym. No dessert for me tonight! Hey, speaking of food . . . I'm kinda hungry. I wonder what we're ordering for lunch*), brush them gently aside and redirect your attention to the area where you left off. You might also deliberately soften or relax each of these areas as you investigate sensations along the way.

As if you've never noticed these areas before (and maybe you haven't!), scan through the lower, middle, and upper back and shoulders, arms, wrists, and hands. Next, turn your attention to the belly, chest, neck and throat, jaw, cheeks, lips, mouth, and tongue. Bring awareness to the eyes, brow, forehead, and scalp. Then notice the body in its entirety, seated and calm(er). Now usher this embodied awareness into the next part of your workday, returning your attention to your slightly more familiar body at any time.

Adapt the Desk Body Scan to fit the amount of time you have available to you (anywhere from a brief thirty-second scan to a more leisurely five-minute break), your surroundings (sitting at your desk at work, in your car in the parking lot, or lying down in bed at home), and your level of privacy. (In more open work spaces, you can sit quietly with eyes open for a moment or two and no one will be the wiser. In fact, they may mistake your mindful break for deep, pensive work-related brainstorming, which in reality it might lead to.) Over time you will more readily notice subtle body sensations as well as become more acquainted with your unique stress signature areas. Use this information wisely, honoring the messages your body is sending you. Pause. Slow down. Pay attention. Stretch. Rest. Move. Breathe. Your body *and mind* will thank you.

Kindness

*If you have good thoughts, they will shine out of your face
like sunbeams and you will always look lovely.*

—Roald Dahl

"I hate people." Regardless of how many times I hear someone utter this powerful phrase, I feel unsettled and completely caught off guard. This negatively charged statement causes me to involuntarily sit up straight in my chair because, at my core, I just cannot fathom it. Sure, people can frustrate, hurt, and anger me, but I believe the vast majority of us are doing the best we can. And though I understand that many who proclaim their hatred are simply attempting to express frustration or erroneously believe it will protect their heart from hurt, this pessimistic worldview carries unnecessarily harmful consequences by keeping them stuck in a defensive, narrow, unhelpful posture.

This type of cynicism can also show up as a temporary symptom of burnout. When we are living in a state of time scarcity and overwhelm, we lose sight of our values and need for connection, and other humans can begin to feel like distractions and stressful obligations.

Our beliefs are powerful in that we unknowingly morph thoughts into facts. We also unconsciously search our environment for evidence for further proof that our beliefs are true. If we are holding firm that "people suck" (another one that raises my hackles), we will certainly find evidence to back up that claim. Conversely, if we believe people are innately good, we will encounter more validation to fill up that bucket of beliefs. I would much rather live in a world with benevolent folks. Fortunately, our mindset around this is largely under our control. Regardless of our overall worldview of humanity, with brief practices we can shift it more toward the positive.

Research backs up this assertion. According to Barbara Fredrickson, a professor who researches positive emotion, and her team, kindness meditation increases our daily perception of positive emotions. When we experience more positivity, research shows, we are more receptive to social support, remain healthier, and strengthen our mindfulness and purpose in life. Overall, these benefits promote increased life satisfaction and a reduction in depression.[6] Not only that, but according to another study, in the journal *Emotion*, just a few minutes of kindness meditation raise both conscious and unconscious feelings of positivity and social connection toward the chosen recipients.[7]

It is certainly more challenging to summon and bestow kindness when we are busy or overwhelmed, but with this quick mindful break, we can usher some feel-good, contagious compassion into any part of our day.

The Kindness Mindful Break

Wherever you are, look around, choose two people randomly, and quietly think, *I wish for this person to be happy. I wish for that person to be happy.* Chade-Meng Tan, author of *Search Inside Yourself* and former mindfulness pioneer at Google, teaches this deceivingly simple *ten-second* exercise as a surefire happiness booster.

❶ Sit for a few minutes with eyes open or closed, wishing happiness for yourself. Allow that intention to assimilate.

❷ Next, choose someone for whom it's easy to send kindness, a loved one or good friend, and wish this person happiness. Notice any body sensations that arise as you do. Imagine how they might feel receiving it.

❸ Now, choose a neutral person, someone you don't know well. Wish them happiness.

❹ If you are feeling brave, choose a somewhat difficult person and send them this kindness, reminding yourself that this person, like you, really just wants to be happy. If you observe resistance or tightening in the body, take a deep breath and relax those muscles. This is a gentle practice not meant to be forced.

❺ Finally, imagine wishing happiness for all people in the world, including yourself, sending it as far and wide as you would like to imagine. Do this every day for a week and watch your capacity for kindness and compassion expand.

Keeping Panic at Bay

It's hard to breathe; the air is hot, stagnant. I look around frantically at the other passengers packed tightly in the old train car. A young mother attempts to open a window in vain, able to budge it only a crack. No matter. In the midst of this Paris summer heat wave, the air outside is just as thick, oppressive, and oxygen-deprived as it is inside. The sweltering humidity bears down upon us, sweat slowly beading up before sliding down my face, neck, chest, and back. Over the crackling overhead speaker, the conductor announces what we've already surmised—a delayed departure.

My fellow travelers become increasingly restless, wipe wet brows, and shift uneasily in narrow seats, their discomfort leaning threateningly toward desperation. I glimpse it in the eyes of the college-age backpacker seated across from me, so close his knees nearly touch mine, and in the young mother's fruitless fanning of her little one. I peer over at my seventeen-year-old daughter and watch nervously as her eyes grow wide, my mind quickly registering her expression—she is teetering on the precipice of a full-blown panic attack. In a whispered voice, I firmly instruct her to close her eyes and take deep breaths, lengthening each exhale. I reassure her that we will be on our way soon and hope I sound more convincing than I feel, for I, too, am struggling.

At a primal, maternal level, I intuit that she is depending on me to remain calm and steady for us both. I close my eyes and fall back on the meditation practice with which I've begun my mornings for the last fourteen years. I ease my shoulders downward, unknit my brow, and observe the natural rising and falling of my lower abdomen. *Inhale. Exhale. Rising. Falling.* My attention darts to the prominent feeling of pressure in my chest. I notice and, as best I can, accept the current body sensations as they are. I usher my attention back to the rising and falling of my belly. Inhale. Exhale. I wonder, *When will this end?* I imagine the sweet relief of cool air. *It's okay*, I coax myself. *Inhale, exhale.* Rivulets of sweat repeatedly usurp my tenuous attention. *Notice. Allow. Breathe.*

Slowly, the panicky feelings subside, moving out like the tide. My strength is restored. I open my eyes to check on my daughter, who, with eyes still closed, seems to have steadied herself as well. The train sputters and rolls away from the station and a rush of air circulates blissfully through the cracked windows. We all breathe a deep, collective sigh of relief.

Mindfulness has come to my rescue on numerous occasions—during post-partum depression, while watching loved ones in pain, and in overwhelming moments of conflict, fear, and grief. Though my Paris tale may be a first-world, privileged problem of sorts, it is also a real-life illustration of mindfulness's powerful grounding effects. Whether faced with the all-encompassing pain of loss or merely withstanding a temporarily unpleasant situation, the Keeping Panic at Bay Mindful Break is a steadying anchor of calm in any life-storm.

The Keeping Panic at Bay Mindful Break

A lot is unknown to us these days; our illusion of control has dissolved. Now more than ever, we need to breathe deeply in order to calm ourselves and our collective fear, to bolster our ability to ride out the discomfort. Without a relatively calm body and mind, not much is possible. Only then can we take steps forward, achieve small goals, and build healthy habits so as not to get stuck in overwhelm.

❶ Notice
Close your eyes, if possible, though this break can be practiced with eyes open. Starting with the feet and moving upward, briefly scan through each section of the body—lower legs, upper legs, bottom, stomach, chest, lower back, upper back—noticing and relaxing any areas of tension. Drop the shoulders, allow the arms to hang loosely, and soften the hands. Relax the jaw and tongue. Unfurrow the brow and forehead. Along the way, you might recognize other sensations not so easily mitigated, such as heaviness in the chest, nausea, aching muscles, headache, or stomachache. Simply notice.

❷ Allow

When faced with unpleasantness, fierce resistance is common in both body and mind. Muscles tighten and futile thoughts implore: *Why is this happening? This is so horrible! I can't do this!* The more we resist, the more painful it is, as we heap on the layers of struggle. Allowing does not mean giving up or giving in; it means acknowledging conditions as they are *in this moment*. Of course, if something can be done to immediately alleviate the suffering, by all means, do. If, however, you have little control (except over your reaction), *lean in to allowing*. Though you may not like it one bit, it *is* your current reality. As best you can, allow and accept, for now.

❸ Breathe

When we are in distress, we unconsciously, intermittently hold our breath and breathe shallowly in the chest, alerting our nervous system to a threat. In order to counteract a cascade of fight-or-flight reactions, breathe deeply, filling up the belly and chest on the inhale and emptying on the exhale. Allowing the breath to come and go in its own rhythm, bring your attention to the natural rising and falling in the belly. When your attention drifts off, as it surely will, kindly and firmly return it to the home base of the breath. Begin again and again, as you patiently ride out the passing storm.

Notice. Allow. Breathe. May the Keeping Panic at Bay Mindful Break serve you well on this ever-changing adventure of life.

Oxygen

We can only be said to be alive in those moments when
our hearts are conscious of our treasures.

—Thornton Wilder

In my psychotherapy office hangs a photograph my brother
took as a college student studying abroad during his junior
year. Shades of burgundy and gold outline the yellow orb of light
descending toward the black-sand beaches of Santorini, Greece,
at sunset. The image soothes me, perhaps out of a sense of nostal-
gia, having visited that very beach three years before my brother
(now a lifetime ago), and also for its natural, simplistic beauty.
Intentionally positioned across from the couch on which my clients settle in for sessions, it is a tranquil balm for them as well.

I chose this photo to decorate my office without giving much
thought to its evidence-based calming abilities, save my own personal experience. It was then remarkable to find studies suggest-
ing that by immersing ourselves in nature, even for short periods
of time, we reduce stress.[9] Even more amazing, we experience
similar benefits by simply *viewing* images of the natural world.

As a lover of the outdoors, this is not at all surprising to me. How satisfying to see my intuition backed up by scientific research!

Of course, depending on where you were raised, where you now reside, and how often you commune with Mother Nature (if ever), this may be either shocking or totally obvious to you. Whether you are a city mouse or a country mouse, soaking up the natural world is good for your overall mental, physical, emotional, and spiritual health.

Based on your workplace and employee culture, there may be a cadre of colleagues who quietly migrate every few hours to the nearest designated outdoor area. I propose that we all use this time to partake in twice-daily Oxygen Mindful Breaks. Whether or not you are drawn to the outdoors, there is a lot to be said for stepping outside and to be reminded that there is a much larger world out there. Broadening our perspective is powerful, adding in some oxygen-rich fresh air and nature, even more so. According to research by Robin Mejia, journalist and professor at Carnegie Mellon University, the first five minutes outside has the most substantial benefit.[10]

In an ideal world, your office building includes enormous windows that allow plenty of sunlight to stream in and are open to unobstructed views of lush greenery and a variety of birds, chipmunks, and other forms of wildlife, with outdoor walking paths and picnic areas. Even better, you work within short strolling distance of a modest patch of woods. As one Japanese study indicates, "Forest environments promote lower concentrations of cortisol, lower pulse rate, lower blood pressure, greater para-sympathetic nerve activity, and lower sympathetic nerve activity than do city environments." Those who regularly access wooded areas experience a decrease in stress hormones, more efficient digestion, a slower heart rate, and a reduction in the triggering of the fight-or-flight response.[11]

Most of us are not so lucky. Our offices vary wildly and there may be little fresh air available, especially if you work in an urban setting. No worries, as I've got a variation of this mindful break for all of us. Fortunately, we can derive similar health benefits from gazing at the natural world through a window. As Florence Williams, environment, health, and science writer, reports in *National Geographic* magazine, "Measurements of stress hormones, respiration, heart rate, and sweating suggest that short doses of nature—or even pictures of the natural world—can calm people down and sharpen their performance."

Go ahead and savor an image or photograph of nature. This pause—any engagement with nature—not only reduces stress but also contributes to more overall calmness and kindness, as well. As Williams goes on to note, "Korean researchers used functional MRI to watch brain activity in people viewing different images. When the volunteers were looking at urban scenes, their brains showed more blood flow in the amygdala, which processes fear and anxiety. In contrast, the natural scenes lit up the anterior cingulate and the insula—areas associated with empathy and altruism."[12]

The Oxygen Mindful Break can be literal—go outside—or imagined—savor a nature scene through a window or with your favorite photograph. By slowing down a notch and soaking up nature's healing effects, you will return to work with increased engagement and a wider, more balanced, perspective.

The Oxygen Mindful Break

Where? First identify where you will go for your oxygen break at work. Count yourself lucky if you have a nature-filled area accessible in proximity. Your break may consist of stepping outside your ten-story building in the middle of a bustling city and gazing upward in order to access a sliver of blue sky. Or maybe you locate a window offering a view of the clouds, a tree, or wildflowers. If you don't have access to either of these scenic possibilities, a nature-filled image will do just fine. Find a photo to use as your screen saver for a momentary break. Change it up to keep it fresh and noticeable to your eye as you log in each morning.

When? Start with two Oxygen Breaks per workday. Ideally, one in the morning and one in the afternoon. Identify when you will take them, remembering that new routines are most easily ingrained if we bookend them between two already established habits. Set up a reminder with sticky notes, phone pings, or planned times in the day.

How? Stop and take a few deep breaths, closing your eyes if you'd like. Listen to the sounds all around, near and far, natural and manmade. If you are gazing out a window or at a photograph, imagine sounds that would accompany your scene if you were immersed in it. Open your eyes and take in the view as if you've never seen it before. Notice colors, textures, shadow, and light. What draws your eye? Is there movement in the form of plant life or critters?

Try enlisting a colleague to keep you accountable and make it fun. Find someone who won't think you've lost your mind for gazing at a photograph of the Grand Canyon. You can show her this mindful break for proof of your still-intact sanity and the research accompanying it.

Take it further. Especially if you are a city dweller, take to the woods after work or on the weekend. If you are insistent on your disdain for all things bugs, dirt, and nature, I encourage you (double dare you) to give walking outdoors a try. Take in the sights, sounds, and scents. If you are feeling especially badass, challenge yourself with a hike. You just might discover some unexpected peace in the process. And if you are a nature lover who has not been out for a hike in years, let this mindful break serve as a reminder of that lost outdoor love. Ink it into your schedule now.

Tracking Your Energy

Every day of our lives, we are on the verge of making those slight changes that would make all the difference.
—Mignon McLaughlin

You know the heavy-bodied, mind-numbing, yet satisfying and blissful exhaustion that ensues after the completion of an intense months-long project or nail-biting end-of-the-quarter meeting? That is *exactly* how I feel when wrestling with client health insurance benefits for my psychotherapy practice—except, of course, for the blissful and satisfied part. The mere thought of calling and navigating the intricate, impassible automated prompt system that renders it impossible to connect with a human being makes me want to curl up in the fetal position among the pillows on my office couch, slipping quickly into in a delightful, protracted nap—an insurance coma, of sorts. Regardless of what type of work you do, I am sure you can relate, as we all have, to at least a few aspects of our work and home lives that completely drain us and that we would rather *never* have to deal with again.

Most of us would love to increase our overall energy level and the ability to sustain it. While I have met the occasional woman who suffers from an *overabundance* of energy (typically driven by anxiety or caffeine), hers is not the ideal as it is unendurable over the long haul. And though we might acknowledge how our stamina is impacted by our stress level, amount of quality sleep, and the food we consume, we are not always aware of how our various daily responsibilities affect our levels of energy. Some tasks are energy suckers, depleting us of mental and physical vigor, while others are energy boosters, fueling our spirit, enhancing our performance, and promoting overall growth. Thankfully, we can learn to add, subtract, and delegate accordingly.

Within the work realm, I find myself most alive when collaborating with and/or mentoring others; writing (only once I've overcome the daily resistance and found my groove); being immersed in an engaging psychotherapy session; teaching mindfulness workshops; and hearing from those who have successfully incorporated mindfulness into their lives through my teaching. Independent of work, I am energized by playing outside in nearly any form—walking, running, biking, kayaking, gardening—either solo, with a friend, or with my family; blissfully perusing the library stacks and diving into a good book; cuddling up to read with my six-year-old son; and chatting with my daughter and husband about life in general.

On the other hand, the work chores I find most draining are insurance billing for client sessions, writing detailed reports, and therapy with the rare unmotivated client. On the home front, a few of my kid's favorite pastimes—creating LEGO constructions and watching mind-numbing video games—bore me to tears.

There are also tasks that fall into a neutral category, such as the laundry, which I find to be neither energizing nor draining. Some neutral chores can take on a more positive, possibly even energizing, tone when mindfulness is brought to them.

There is also a subtle but critical distinction between feeling depleted and feeling tired but knowing that your time has been well used. For example, I love the exhausting but pleasing muscle fatigue one gets from gardening or shoveling snow. Likewise, when five o'clock Friday afternoon hits, after a full week of client appointments, I am mentally spent but in the best possible way. My family knows that Friday evenings I likely won't have much capacity for conversation. It is a contented, purposeful tiredness, as opposed to feeling drained. This balance could easily sway into the realm of total depletion if I attempt to see too many clients per day or allow my ongoing self-care to fall by the wayside.

Now pause for a moment and consider how *you* would describe your energy level these days. Perhaps you are tense, exhausted, and running on nothing but fumes by the end of the workweek. Maybe the tiredness is more subtle, consisting of a modest yet pervasive sense of fatigue. Even if you are mostly content, you can still benefit from tuning in to the more subtle variations in energy in order to protect and maintain that sweet spot of balance.

Using your trusty sense of recollection, conjure up your most recent relaxing vacation. (If you scan through the memory files and come up blank, oh boy, you are without a doubt overdue. Go schedule yourself some time off this instant and/or head to the Play Hooky Mindful Break, page 235.) Recall your sense of mental and physical energy at the tail end of your time off. You were most likely feeling tranquil yet alert, with a sustained amount of get-up-and-go. Now juxtapose this with your typical amount of work energy. Can you imagine sustaining your current career pace for the next five to ten years? This renders some women deer-in-the-headlights shocked—body frozen, eyes wide in alarm—when contemplating this thought.

Day after day we push ahead with the unconscious assumption that the current chaos is temporary when, in fact, if no conscious changes are made, we will undoubtedly find ourselves in the exact same position five years down the road (unless illness or burnout hits first). While it may be a reach to expect that work feels as peaceful as our favorite vacation, we can (and should) tweak our current conditions to bring a bit of that restful calm to our work day.

Of course, there are plenty of external, at times unavoidable, factors that influence our energy, such as sleep quantity and quality, illness, caregiving responsibilities, loss, and other life stressors. Our levels naturally wax and wane throughout the day. Without a doubt, though, what we choose to spend our time on matters and plays a significant role in our feeling either completely burned out or ready to tackle the world.

The Tracking Your Energy Mindful Break

In this mindful break you will learn a number of ways to bring focused attention to what lights you up and what depletes you. Experiment with one method at a time, remaining curious about the information it provides. Mentally note your observations or record them in a notebook or phone, either throughout the day or at the end of it. If you want to dive into a more extensive version of this break, you can document your time through an entire week or month in half-hour increments, noting which activities energize (+), deplete (-), or are perceived as neutral (0).

❶ As you wake in the morning mentally run through the day's schedule. Take an inner snapshot of each upcoming activity, distinguishing between which aspects prompt a bored, tired sigh and which you anticipate with excitement. Notice the accompanying body sensations for each. Are your back and shoulders tense? Are you inhaling shallowly in the chest rather than taking full, relaxed belly breaths? Or is your body at ease—alert and eager to greet the day? As you hone your attention in this way, you may recognize how your energy level is affected not only by tasks but also by other factors, such as people or your own thoughts. (Hold on to this information, which can be applied to Your Inner Bully, page 140, and Challenging People Mindful Breaks, page 212.)

❷ As you go about your day, familiarize yourself with how each of your activities contributes to or detracts from your energy. While transitioning from one task to another, notice which are the energy suckers, which light you up, and which seem more neutral. Though an energizing task might require concentration, it also has an effortless quality, perhaps even exponentially multiplying our vigor. Depleting activities leave us exhausted and mentally spent. Neutral has more of a *meh,* flat quality to it; we can take it or leave it.

❸ Now identify what, specifically, in the depleting list might be removed or delegated. If it seems as if nothing could possibly fit this bill, take a deep breath and examine those tasks again, this time with a more detached, open-minded perspective. There is always something that can be adjusted, however minimal doing so might first appear. Take note of what old habits or outdated narratives may be keeping you stuck. You may want to enlist a trusted friend whose more objective view can help bring possible modifications to light.

It's common to feel resistance as you consider relinquishing control of a long-held (if even long-despised) task. You may fear upsetting the status quo or find it difficult to trust that the necessary resources are in place. I, too, have struggled with these self-imposed barriers—and I'm happy to report that after a number of years I have finally delegated all insurance company billing to my wonderful assistant. Those fetal-position naps on my office couch are now gratefully a thing of the past. And let me tell you, *it feels amazing.* My time and mental energy can now be spent on things that fully engage me, such as, well, writing this book. Change is almost universally uncomfortable. Thankfully, we humans accommodate and adapt remarkably fast. Rest easy in the knowledge that the early discomfort is temporary. Be patient and encouraging with yourself.

If farming out responsibilities requires financial resources not currently at your disposal, you might find a way to barter services or designate it as part of your long-term plan. A few years back I promised myself that when my younger child started full-time school, which allowed me to schedule a few extra clients per month, I would hire a billing administrator. Reminding myself of the future plan periodically helped soften the unpleasant edges of my weekly insurance billing tasks.

When it comes to delegating, transferring even the most seemingly minimal tasks to someone else can dramatically lighten our mental and physical energy load. Handing over the grocery shopping to your spouse, mobilizing the older children for ongoing household chores, or asking a colleague to take an unpleasant (to you, not necessarily to them) task off your plate can free up precious energy.

Of course not all work tasks are under our control. When you have determined that certain responsibilities cannot be removed from your list, it is time to shift your *attitude* toward them. After all, our perspective is totally under our control. Rather than tighten up—physically, with tense muscles, or mentally, with negative thoughts or verbal complaints—we can attend to these unpleasant tasks mindfully, with a sense of curiosity and compassion for ourselves, and with full acknowledgment that it is a depleting yet necessary task.

❹ Finally, I offer the reminder that sprinkling our days with all sorts of mindful breaks helps sustain energy longer, either by calming (such as the Wide-Awake Mindful Break, page 119), connecting (Kindness, page 55) or invigorating (the Afternoon Slump, page 178). There is no need to act on the data you acquire all at once. Keep the attitude light, experimental, and playful. Take your time, as this is a lifelong practice meant to be freely recalibrated over and over again.

ShondaLand

———

*Where we think we need more self-discipline, we usually
need more self-love—not just self-love as an attitude, but
self-love manifested through the routines and rituals that
we set up to enable the changes we desire to happen
naturally and with ease.*

—Tara Mohr

The ShondaLand Mindful Break owes its name to my funny,
insightful client Christine, who happens to be endowed not
only with a flair for the dramatic but also with a prolific amount
of self-judgment regarding recent life transitions and growing
pains. Dealing with anxiety and overwhelm, Christine needed
some fast-acting calming techniques to pull her swirling mind
and jittery body back down to Earth.

I instructed Christine to place her hands over her heart as
a physical reminder to release the persistent worry and self-
judgment, come back to her breath, and offer herself some reassuring kindness. This simple exercise releases oxytocin, the
calming hormone promoting safety and trust. It is grounding,
soothing, and accessible to us at any moment.

Christine, not shy about spilling the contents of our meetings with a handful of close friends, shared the hands-to-heart practice with them. Collectively, they began referring to our sessions as "going to ShondaLand." (For those of you not in the know, Shonda Rhimes, creator of *Grey's Anatomy*, television producer, screenwriter, and author, ends her TV show credits with an image of ShondaLand.)

Now, when Christine reaches out to those friends in a moment of struggle, they implore her to *go to ShondaLand*, code for placing hands on heart and breathing deeply, eliciting a giggle in addition to that much-needed sense of peace. I was both amused and touched when Christine shared this with me. I am offering this self-compassionate mindful break so you, too, can go to ShondaLand anytime, anywhere.

The ShondaLand Mindful Break

1 Recognize the need for some calm, self-kindness, or healthy self-soothing.

2 Place both hands over your heart, noticing the sensation of touch, warmth, and the feel of your heartbeat.

3 Take a few full inhales and exhales, bringing your attention to the area of the chest as it rises and falls with the breath.

4 Repeat, either softly or silently, a calming phrase or word. "You're OK, you're OK." "Calm, calm," or "This, too, shall pass." Experiment until you hit upon something that resonates.

5 Share this powerful mindful break with your loved ones, in whatever form your little heart desires.

Waiting

———

We can be sure that the greatest hope for maintaining equilibrium in the face of any situation rests within ourselves.

—Francis J. Braceland

Oh, the wai-ai-ting is the hardest part . . . especially if you are a (recovering) type A like me. Patience is not my finest virtue. Thanks in part to my mindfulness practice, it is an area in which I have undoubtedly improved but nevertheless have a way to go. On any given day, I can slip easily, nearly imperceptibly, into hyperproductivity mode, each item enthusiastically crossed off the list with a flourish. When I move at this rapid pace, I automatically anticipate the same level of efficiency from my unsuspecting environs, my trusty computer included. Which is how I found myself at the close of a particularly engrossing psychotherapy session growing frustrated with the achingly sluggish pace of my electronic records scheduling system. Waiting with my client for the program to load in order to book our next appointment, I sighed emphatically, bemoaning the (horror!) full ninety-second wait, a therapeutic model of mindfulness and patience. Ahem.

We are all a work in progress, including the mindfulness coach herself. Part of the fun of mindfulness is finding amusement and self-compassion in our foibles rather than judging ourselves for our very unmindful reactions. Life presents endless opportunities to try again, and none of us gets it right all the time. Thankfully, mindfulness is also very forgiving.

As far as my computer woes, I wish I could report that I quickly realized the error of my intolerant ways, but alas, only after reacting impatiently a number of times did I recognize I had a choice in my response: I could continue with the fruitless sighing complaints or I could use the opportunity for a much more beneficial Waiting Mindful Break.

The Waiting Mindful Break

Whenever you find yourself a captive audience—as you wait for a meeting to begin, in line at the grocery store, or while your computer is loading—instead of compulsively checking e-mail, complaining, or scrolling through social media once again, make mindful use of your time. As you begin, you may be shocked to recognize the frequency and urgency with which you automatically, unconsciously, reach for your phone. Don't panic. That magnetic pull you feel toward being connected 24-7 is common and completely adjustable. The first step to modifying any behavior is bringing it into full awareness, including, in this case, the powerful discomfort of resisting a peek.

Start by taking a few long, deep inhales and exhales, bringing your full attention to each breath. Next, scan your body beginning with the head to notice where you are holding tension. Soften the small muscles around the eyes, the brow, the mouth, the jaw. Allow the shoulders to drop (I sometimes find mine up in the vicinity of my ears) and the arms to hang from the shoulders. Soften the muscles in the back, belly, and legs. Your attention might wander once again to your phone or some other distraction. This is not a problem. Simply note the urge and once again direct your attention back to the breath. Notice you are alive and breathing. Let this be a brief time where nothing needs to be done, solved, fixed, or planned.

I kindly challenge you to be on the lookout for waiting opportunities wherever you can uncover them. You can take a thirty-second Waiting Mindful Break or stretch it out for a few minutes. Be patient with yourself; you are relearning how to slow down and simply *be* for a short time. This does not always feel initially pleasant, but if you remain curious, it often changes with a bit of practice. Eventually, you might even welcome the chance to wait, slow down, and take a much-needed Waiting Mindful Break.

Bathroom

Tara, a fortysomething elementary school administrator, wife, and mom, reached out to me in hopes of curtailing the stress and overwhelm that had reached a fever pitch in her life. Conscientious and perfectionistic, Tara continually put others before herself. She was often drawn into her colleagues' dramatic, fruitless crises before recognizing what hit her, and she regularly stayed long after hours in order to accommodate their top-priority projects. It was no surprise that her tolerance was low, patience worn thin, and resentment growing by the day.

Tara described colleagues frantically flitting about the office, inundated with paperwork and meetings, affecting and infecting each other's negative moods. Starting with five minutes of guided meditation each morning, Tara was more able to tune in to the nuances of her stress and overwhelm, especially at work. Tasting a bit of tranquility while meditating, she soon began craving bits of calm while embroiled in the nonstop activity of her day. Together, we set about determining which mindful breaks would fit seamlessly into her particular work environment.

Several times a week, Tara visits a handful of schools, where there is no private office space, and a constant stream of staff jockeys for a few moments of her time. As is the case for many of us, Tara is not in the advantageous position of being able to close her own office door and hide—I mean, carve out a moment of quiet time for herself. The challenge lay in *where* to carve out a private moment, in addition to when.

After some brainstorming, we hit upon the perfect solution . . . drumroll, please . . . Tara would be taking her much-needed mindful breaks in the lovely staff bathroom. Not the classiest of options, but functional. You gotta do whatcha gotta do to take care of yourself, often requiring creativity, flexibility, and, shall we say, open-mindedness?

So, when Tara began to feel the tension in her shoulders or her mind swimming with thoughts, she'd politely excuse herself and head straight for the restroom, where she'd lock the door, take a few deep breaths, stretch, and regroup. Though not her optimal Zen choice, it was a brief opportunity to step out of the chaos so prevalent in her surroundings.

With a few weeks of daily meditation and special bathroom breaks under Tara's belt, her family and work friends started to notice a positive difference in her ability to pause, take a breath, and assess if there truly was a crisis rather than automatically diving in with the rest of them. Tara has observed an increase in her physical and emotional stamina. Best of all, she is once again smiling, laughing, and enjoying work and home. Tara joked that she feels like the female version of Clark Kent, ducking into the staff bathroom and emerging as Mindful Superwoman. Who knew a few stolen moments and a Bathroom Mindful Break would lead to such mighty superpowers?

The Bathroom Mindful Break

❶ Location, location, location. If the lack of private work space challenges your ability to steal a few quiet moments for yourself, conjure up the best possible solution amid your current conditions. At work, this might look like a utility closet, little-used stairwell, or bathroom.

❷ Zone in. Pause, stand up tall, and take a few slow, deep breaths. As best you can, bring your attention to immediate body sensations, leaving the chaos of work on the other side of that door.

❸ Stretch it out. If you can spare a few more moments, move and stretch various body parts from head to toe.

❹ Talk yourself down. If you are fleeing from a particularly stressful situation, you might repeat a calming, grounding phrase. *This, too, is passing. You've got this. One thing at time.*

❺ Exit strategy. Before joining the fray once again, check your posture—stand tall, shoulders back. Keep breathing. You've got this. Go get 'em.

Meetings

Calm is contagious.
                                                            —Rorke Denver

After a few months of her own personal mindfulness practice, Tara, of Bathroom Mindful Break, noticing how stressed out her colleagues were, decided to slowly introduce the concept of mindfulness into her workplace. With a spirit of experimentation mixed with confident resolve, Tara decided to start with a short practice in a small staff meeting. Having described most of her colleagues as either distracted and disengaged or high-strung and stressed out, Tara's hope was that the meetings would become more efficient and engaging yet allow room for collegial connection. She hoped these benefits would translate into the staff's overall work and personal lives, just as mindfulness had for her.

Tara began with a short explanation of mindfulness, its benefits, and how she had personally noticed positive changes in her life as a result of it. As expected, there were a few resistant skeptics. Tara made it clear that, though the mindfulness practice was not mandatory, the quiet and respect for those who chose to partake was. She played a short guided meditation to start their meeting. To her surprise, each person in the room sat quietly for those two minutes, some fidgeting, others stock-still, most revealing afterward how good it felt to uncharacteristically stop for a short time. Later, Tara shared with me that the one person she anticipated would be most antagonistic turned out to be the most receptive of all, which is exactly what I find in trainings. Though we may think we know our colleagues well, it's best to introduce mindfulness with an open mind, as it is impossible to anticipate who will take to it.

As of this writing, still in the midst of integrating mindfulness into her meetings, Tara's proverbial jury is still out regarding its far-reaching benefits, though her colleagues' responses have been overwhelmingly positive. This, combined with her own personally perceived meditation and mindful break success, keep her motivated and intent on offering and supporting mindfulness for all.

Of course, depending on your organizational culture, your formulation of a mindful meeting will vary. Mindful meetings can run the gamut from one big, deep breath before beginning to an organization-wide practice of daily meditation in a dedicated mindfulness space, or anything in between. If you work in a cutting-edge, hip office, meetings might begin with a leisurely five-minute guided meditation followed by colleague check-ins, à la the workplace at Eileen Fisher.

However, if your work culture is such that the mere mention of the word *mindfulness* causes your colleagues to gaze at you as if you'd sprouted an extra head, then your mindful meetings, at least for the time being, might consist of those solo mindful breaks. If going it alone, you can conduct your own one-woman mindful meeting right in the middle of your colleagues' routinely disorganized one. No, I am not recommending you close your eyes and tune them out (though you may fantasize about it), but rather, at the outset, take some deep breaths, drop your shoulders, relax your jaw, and redirect your attention back to the task at hand whenever you've noticed it has wandered off. You'll be surprised by how few seconds it takes to accomplish this. If we work with a resistant crew, sometimes the best we can do is strengthen our own practice, modeling the calm and efficiency it cultivates. It is not necessary to share your personal mindfulness tools if the milieu is not one of open-mindedness and support.

The Meetings Mindful Break

❶ **Do a little office recon.** What does a typical office meeting now look like? Are your coworkers focused and engaged or distracted and bored? Are they rushing from one meeting to another, without a moment to digest or prepare? Guzzling coffee and munching mindlessly on snacks?

❷ **Consider the possibilities.** Imagine how differently everyone would function if encouraged to pause, take a few deep breaths, relax tense muscles, regroup, and bring their full attention to the topics at hand. The power of stopping in the midst of the chaos is often mind-blowing and a huge productivity booster.

❸ Back it up with evidence. If your colleagues are unsure but curious about mindfulness in the workplace, I recommend explaining the research and rationale behind it (see Resource Guide, page 277).

❹ Use a guide. Ideally, hire a mindfulness coach who can guide your organization, returning for follow-up sessions to maintain momentum, progress, and accountability while helping colleagues negotiate any practice hurdles that arise. If you have a willing crew but no trainer in the prescribed budget, you can also utilize an app or online resource to guide the brief meditation.

If you are lucky enough to work in an office that has been millennially Google-ized, *mindfulness* is a frequently used word, and just about everyone is up for it. You've got it easy and can simply use this book to support your already mindful work culture.

❺ Tailor it to your unique workplace. Perhaps you add colleague check-ins, in which each person briefly shares the general state of her life, both at home and at work, at the outset of each meeting. If so, establish basic ground rules so the well-meaning office Chatty Cathy does not unknowingly usurp all the allotted time and cause the meeting to run over. As uncomfortable and initially unpopular as it may be, explicitly state and guard the expectation that all distracting devices are shut off for meetings.

⑥ Be persistent and patient. Consistency is key. Before long, your team will expect and anticipate those few moments of welcome quiet, regrouping, and regained focus.

Lunch

Slowing down is a power move.   **—Amy Cuddy**

We all know that dedicated career-driven women never waste time on a proper lunch break, right? Unconsciously scarfing down a sandwich in five minutes flat while fully absorbed in the task at hand demonstrates not only a zealous, enviable work ethic but also the ultimate in productivity. Even better is consuming no lunch at all, save the random two Oreos eaten on the way to a meeting (followed by a hasty mouth swish of water to erase any trace of guilty chocolate remains, of course). However ludicrous sounding when penned on the page, this is an all-too-familiar scene. How many of us have bought into the concept of a no-time-to-waste midday feeding frenzy in some form? I know that more than once I have been guilty as charged.

Skipping meals, for me, is a completely foreign concept. I am among those humans whose mood can mutate from pleasantly jovial to downright hangry in a matter of seconds, which is no joke. So, although I am only prone to skipping meals when seriously under the weather, I *am* responsible for devouring some awfully *unmindful* lunches while seated at my office desk. For it is on those days when it seems I don't have a moment to spare that I place the substantial, beautifully colorful salad next to my computer and diligently chomp away at those fresh vegetables, oblivious to their deliciousness. Even more lamentable is when I have packed myself a treat—a piece of tasty dark chocolate or freshly baked cookie—and this, too, goes down the hatch without the least bit of relishing. Focusing intently on returning that e-mail or drafting that article, I barely register having eaten anything at all. Not savoring a salted chocolate chip cookie to the fullest? Now that is an unthinkable disgrace.

Speaking of cookies, just imagine how a cartoon version of ourselves might depict the spectacle of our oblivious munching of those Oreos: Oh yes, incoming!, shout the excited, wide-open eyes as the beloved cookie makes its way to eager lips. The salivating mouth and impatient taste buds let out a quiet, satisfied mmmm as they luxuriate in the crisp yet creamy hunk of tastiness—but for only a split second. That's how long the cookie is allowed to hang out atop the tongue before it swiftly plummets down the startled throat (cough-cough), landing in the stomach (plunk!), which, all morning, has been attempting in vain to capture your attention with assorted grumbles and rumblings.

Finally!, says the relieved stomach, *some long-awaited nourishment! Psych! No real nutrients here, just a huge unmasticated lump of sugar requiring pointless digestive effort.*

Fantastic, laments the brain, *now how will I find the energy to craft any brilliant, creative thoughts?*

We'd like to file a grievance, chime in the rest of your organs. *Frankly, we are sick and tired of the lack of respect for our amazing, ceaseless functioning in spite of inadequate fuel. If our demands for healthy change are not met, we will cease our vigorous function and you will certainly suffer. Maybe not today, perhaps not tomorrow, but we can guarantee the time will come.*

Has the fear- and guilt-inducing message been received loud and clear? Rather than wallow in the shame of neglecting our bodies, heed these words as a benevolent wake-up call. What if we actually regarded and fed our bodies like the miraculous goddesses they are? Regardless of the shape, size, and fitness level of your bod and what you think of her, she relentlessly keeps you functioning at your best. It's time to recognize her overall awesomeness and start feeding her that way.

Essentially, the antidote to skipping meals, inhaling them unconsciously, or overeating is to choose and consume our food mindfully. Mindful eating, simply put, is paying attention to the body's level of hunger, satisfying it with predominantly balanced nutritious food, noticing as we do, and eating until just satisfied.

Don't worry, I am not advocating a strict diet devoid of treats. Oh no, I would never, as someone with an undeniable sweet tooth. I love the pie, the ice cream, the homemade chocolate cake. Life is way too short to deprive myself of all that yumminess. Fortunately, I enjoy mostly veggies, fruit, and other nutritious foods; learning to eat mindfully has helped me get there.

The Lunch Mindful Break

As always, start where you are, beginning with one or two small changes at a time. When appropriate, let your dining companions in on your mindful eating plan, inviting everyone to pause and take a breath with you before diving in.

❶ Pay attention to hunger and satiety (*when* and *how much* you eat). To decide *when* and *how much*, start by assessing your hunger. On a scale of one to ten (one is not at all, ten is ready to gnaw your own arm off, which is the hanger talking), rate your current level of hunger. Ideally, we feed our bodies when we are *between five and seven*. If below five, you are not ready for a meal; if above seven, there is a tendency to overeat or dive into the scary depths of "hangriness." When you are considering eating, pause and notice the accompanying body sensations. Is there a hollowness in the belly? Burning, churning, or slight discomfort? It is important to distinguish between true hunger and an emotion-driven emptiness. Loneliness, anxiety, and boredom can mimic body sensations of hunger. The more we pause and notice regularly, the more easily we can distinguish between the two, realizing just how many extra calories we may have previously been consuming in this barely conscious way.

❷ Follow the 80-20 rule, generally (*what* you choose to eat). We can also learn to stop eating when we are 80 percent full, a practice Okinawans call *hara hachi bun me.*

Maintain awareness throughout the meal so as to determine when you've hit that 80 percent mark, rather than eventually uttering the common, *Ugh, I am so full.* (Hara hachi bun me—not only fun to say but also one of the habits researchers believe contribute to Okinawans' top standing in the world's so-called Blue Zones, regions where the population lives exceptionally long and healthy lives, as written about by Dan Buettner.)

Once you have finished your meal, move your plate out of reach so you are not tempted to continue noshing after you feel satisfied. If you find yourself once again moving toward the plate, pause, and inquire into why. Is it out of boredom, anxiety, or just plain habit? Hara hachi bun me, baby.

Determine *what* to eat by loosely following the 80-20 rule. Eighty percent of your food should be whole, healthy, and nutritious, while the remaining 20 percent is for the empty-calories-but-oh-so-worth-it consumption of the brownie, glass of rosé, or generous hunk of brie.

Whether you disdain anything edible that comes from the earth or have never met a vegetable you don't like, begin with one addition or alteration to your repertoire. If your ratio is flipped 20 percent healthy to 80 not so much, don't overwhelm yourself all at once, as the *eventual* goal is 80 percent. Whether that happens next week or next year, the intention is to maintain this overall ratio in the long run.

❸ Eat mindfully (awareness and enjoyment; support-ing the other two prongs). Eat mindfully with *awareness and enjoyment*: Using your sense of sight, notice the colors and shapes of the food. With gratitude, take a moment to reflect on how the food made its way to the table. Inhale the scents, chewing the first few bites slowly, noticing its temperature and fully tasting flavors and textures. Pay attention to the sensations of swallowing as the food trav-els down your throat.

If eating the entire meal mindfully seems too burden-some, you can focus primarily on the first and last bites, thereby noticing when you have reached the sweet spot of just enough toward the end of the meal. Be sure to savor the infinite variety of foods and methods of preparation available to you. Be adventurous and curious in your eat-ing. Notice your energy level after eating various types of food. You may be surprised at how some can completely sap your energy while others help bolster it for hours. Ulti-mately, mindful eating can tame the growth of our waist-lines and increase sustained energy of both body and mind. You, and your goddess bod, are worth the mindful effort, thought, and attention. Bon appétit and hara hachi bun me.

5-Minute Walk

Dwell on the beauty of life. Watch the stars, and see yourself running with them.

—Marcus Aurelius

B arbara, a full-time career coach who works three days a week in the office and two from home, struggles with blurred lines between work and personal time. In order to transition from one task to another, Barbara created her own version of a mindful break for weather-permitting days when working out of her home office. She told me, "My favorite mindful break when the weather is warm is to walk through the grass in my bare feet. Also known as 'grounding' or 'earthing,' this practice incorporates many senses and is a signal for me to be present. I feel the cool grass, notice the sounds of the outdoors, and smell the fresh air. There is an immediate change in my mood and stress level; I can then return to what I was doing with a new mindset."

Barbara intuitively engages in practices proven to enhance mood and productivity. Research has shown that a fifteen-minute lunchtime walk increases concentration and lessens fatigue throughout the afternoon hours, and it helps us maintain higher levels of well-being at the end of the workday. "These results add to the theory-based knowledge on recovery during workday breaks and highlight the importance of breaks for organizational practices."[13] If you can spare the full fifteen minutes, fantastic. With only five minutes of vigorous walking, though, you will notice the calming, yet energizing shift as well.

The 5-Minute Walk Mindful Break

Schedule your break in advance. It can be challenging to stop what you are doing to take a break if you are happily engaged in workflow. We are more productive and efficient with periodic pauses.

- Get outside. If weather permits, kick off your shoes and feel the cool grass under your feet.

- Move it! Stroll briskly and get your heart pumping, waking up your muscles and mind.

- Notice all the muscles being used for motion, balance, and strength. Consider the countless unconscious actions required for a simple walk.

- If you work from home and have a canine companion, get him in on the action. Barbara also shares that playing fetch with her pooch is another fantastic way to regroup in the midst of a home office workday.

- Though practicing the 5-Minute Walk Mindful Break outdoors is the ideal, it may not be feasible because of weather or office-setting conditions. Climbing a few flights of stairs or a brisk walk around the building, inside or out, can get the heart pumping and prime you for increased alertness, a hit of endorphins, and a boost in confidence.

- After your break, pause to notice the changes in overall body awareness you experience. Are you more mentally alert? Where do you feel increased energy?

- For accountability and high-fives, keep a daily log of your 5-Minute Walk Mindful Breaks. Note where you walked and for how long. What did you notice in your body afterward? How did moving affect your mood for the remainder of your day?

- Get going and enjoy!

Unpleasant Moments

The barn is burned down now. I can see the moon.

—Masahide

Can you guess the life span of an emotion—how long a feeling sticks around after it has arisen? Ninety seconds. Tell that to my emotions, though, because they often act as if they've never received the memo. Ninety seconds. Hard to believe? It was for me, too.

Jill Bolte Taylor, PhD, neuroanatomist and author of *My Stroke of Insight,* found that the natural life span of an emotion is only a minute and a half. In my estimation, this means the average time it takes for an emotion to move through the nervous system and body is about equivalent in length to the intense pain of a drop-you-to-your-knees stub of the toe. Depending on the circumstances, our emotions can feel just as fierce. I find it to be an incredibly comforting and helpful reminder in the midst of an emotional storm that our feelings naturally build, crest, and then abate. We can, after all, tolerate most anything for ninety seconds.

But herein lies the rub. The emotion will subside only if we don't add fuel to the (possibly already raging) fire. In Eastern philosophy this is referred to as shooting the second arrow. The first arrow is the challenge that life hands us—that which is not under our control. The second arrow is shot when we heap additional suffering on top of the original hurt.

Here's an example. As I sat to write one bright winter Sunday afternoon, we in the Northeast were clearing out from a record snowstorm, a blizzard that began Friday evening, slowly abating twenty-four hours later, unloading a whopping thirty inches of snow. With winds at forty miles an hour and temperatures near zero, there was none of the typical frolicking outside during this storm. My family was instead all tucked inside the house together for a fairly long stretch of time. Three of us with colds; one with a (then) four-year-old's infinite amount of energy to burn; one a teenager with little tolerance for said four-year-old's energy; one outside much of the day battling snow with plow and shovel; and one with a looming manuscript deadline. *Gulp*.

You see, I usually spend my Saturdays writing in my quiet therapy office, but I soon altered my expectations of leaving the house upon waking to a foot of snow outside my window. So, after a leisurely breakfast, I retreated to my home office (inconveniently located in the middle of the bustling house), hoping to spend some concentrated time writing. I figured if I could get just two hours in, I'd be able to relax and enjoy the rest of the snowed-in day with my family. A great plan, in theory. However, some hours and countless disruptions later, I was a grumpy, frustrated mess. By midafternoon, I had not written one good coherent sentence, nor had I been fully present with my family at any point throughout the day. I was distracted and unpleasant to be around. I knew it, but I had a hard time stopping it, which only led to more frustration.

The first arrow in this scenario was my inability to find focused writing time amid the pressure of an upcoming deadline, thwarted expectations, and the incessant toggling back and forth between work and family. Somewhat unpleasant, yes, but had I only realized that frustration could be contained to ninety seconds, I could have saved myself hours of futile disgruntlement.

Unfortunately, I didn't catch it in time, thereby automatically shooting the second arrow (and third, fourth, and fifth). The second arrow is the story we tell ourselves about the challenge. It is the dialogue, the judging, and the resistance we add to an already painful situation, and it keeps us stuck in that emotional storm. As I endured interruption after interruption my thoughts sounded something like this: *What is up with this snow? I was so geared up to dive into my work, but clearly that is not happening! How am I going to get this project done on time? No, I do not want to play another round of Monopoly—I want to work! Is that so terrible?!*

And on and on. Although I may not have spoken those actual words aloud, my family received the general message. You get the picture.

Was I being ridiculous and overdramatic? Yes, and we do it all the time. Just watch your mind do its thing the next time a difficulty presents itself. It is a humbling part of the human condition. When we recognize the second arrow, name it, *allow* it (it is already here, so you might as well), and are curious about it, we completely change its hold over us. In retrospect, I should have named the pressure and frustration, noticed it with self-compassion, and then let go of my writing expectations for the day as soon as it was apparent.

> *Suffering equals pain multiplied by resistance.*
> —Shinzen Young

Ninety seconds. No second arrow. So much better.

This is just a minor unpleasant situation in the big scheme of things. But what about those *really* unpleasant moments—the ones that are terrifying, heart wrenching, or rage inducing? How do we work with those? What if it feels too overwhelming? Too intense? Well, fortunately, we work with them in much the same way.

There is always the breath. This is one of the reasons we use the breath as a common point of focus for meditating. It can serve as an anchor for our attention, not to avoid the intense emotions, but to calm ourselves enough so we can face the unpleasant feelings. When we maintain a point of focus, such as on the breath, it allows us to hang on long enough until the difficulty subsides. When we remind ourselves that the intensity will pass if we can breathe, relax our bodies, and stay focused on the inhale and exhale, we have the ability to ride out any emotional storm.

The Unpleasant Moments Mindful Break

If you are facing a minor unpleasantness, be on the lookout for what body sensations tend to arise. Almost like our own little warning system, we each have a unique identifiable pattern that helps us catch what's coming. Can you be aware of your pattern in the future? When you notice unpleasant body sensations arise, bring your full attention to them. Observe the subtleties that compose them, noticing how they change, if they change. While it may not take the unpleasantness away, noticing allows us to pause and choose how we wish to respond to the challenge.

When the situation you are facing is more intense and overwhelming, first remind yourself that if you can gently keep your focus on the body or breath, it will last for only ninety seconds. As best you can, take a few long, deep breaths, relax your body, and bring your attention to the breath. Ground yourself in the feeling of the inhale and exhale. Let it anchor you. Rather than resist the intense emotions, which is often our natural response to something unpleasant, see if you can work on accepting them. Please know that accepting does not equal condoning or inviting. But whether or not we like it, those feelings are here. Can you allow yourself to feel and face them? The more you remain aware and calm, the sooner the storm will pass. You may feel some residual unpleasantness, to be sure, but you will now be more able to tolerate and choose how to respond to it.

Offer yourself plenty of compassion with this mindful break. It is the practice of a lifetime and deserves plenty of patience and respect. May you find comfort in its usefulness. May the second arrow remain untouched in your quiver.

Drowning in Chocolate
(or Too Much
of a Good Thing)

———

Happiness is a place between too much and too little.
—Finnish proverb

The months of November and December are replete with assorted holiday events and festivities, shopping and presents, volunteering and giving, work and family gatherings. With so much of the good stuff happening at once, we can easily descend into an unconscious state of automatic pilot, losing sight of the fortunate nature of all the busyness. As author Dan Harris aptly describes, the overabundance is analogous to "drowning in chocolate," gratefully loving all the celebrations and rituals but overwhelmed nevertheless.

This is a lovely "problem" to have, I realize, and we all fall prey to it. Eventually, though, we face our challenges, a time when we would give anything to be "drowning in chocolate." This mindful break is a friendly reminder to slow down and reconnect with gratitude when we have overextended ourselves and our proverbial cup runneth over; a soft plea (for myself as well as for you) to pause, breathe, pull ourselves out of autopilot, and take time to recognize the abundance so we can savor those precious memories with mindfulness.

When you find yourself spinning out on your wealth of champagne problems, there is no need to judge for losing sight of how good you have it. Rather, consider it the perfect opportunity to notice the ease, the wonderful surplus of "chocolate" in your life right now, and bask in the gratitude.

The Drowning in Chocolate Mindful Break

❶ First congratulate yourself for recognizing that you have fallen into the realm of overabundance and over-scheduling, despite the positive nature of it all.

❷ Take a few deep breaths to calm the body and mind. Allow yourself to return to *this* moment rather than all the upcoming activities in the near future.

❸ Bring attention to your body sensations (relaxed muscles, a smile, a lightness in the chest), emotions (pride, happiness, contentment), and thoughts in order to savor and later remember the moment in its fullness.

❹ Reconnect with gratitude for your good fortune.

Before committing to additional future obligations you

may want to try the Life as Pie Mindful Break, page 230, to avoid overextending yourself.

Be on the lookout for more opportunities to turn off autopilot—especially when things are looking up—and savor. Repeat.

Partners (What Have I Done for You Lately?)

When we focus on our gratitude, the tide of
disappointment goes out and the tide of love rushes in.

—Kristin Armstrong

Want to know the sexiest thing my husband did for me recently? (Now I have your attention!) Nope, he did not sweep me away for a romantic night sans kids, nor did he craft a heartfelt love poem in my honor. My beloved husband spent three and a half hours Saturday morning painstakingly completing my daughter's detailed college financial aid forms. Yup, that's right. If you've not experienced this lovely high school senior rite of passage, suffice it to say it resembles filing income taxes, but a lot less fun. I cannot express how wonderful it felt to have this onerous task taken off my plate.

Why include a mindful break about partners in *Don't Forget to Breathe*? If our home lives are unhappy, conflicted, or distant, it is nearly impossible to shake off the residual effects as we move into the work part of our day. Tolerance and patience diminish, emotional and mental energy are expended on the conflict, and thoughts inevitably drift back home as we attempt to concentrate at work. Sure, to some degree we may be able to compartmentalize, leaving the partner issues at home, especially when focused intently on a project at the office. For the most part, though, a healthy, happy partnership allows us not only to bring our best, most productive selves to work but also to enjoy a more connected, contented home life, and, ultimately, better overall work–life balance.

This particular good deed earned my husband serious brownie points, a back massage, and a four-pack of his favorite IPA from the local brewery. He did remark that he'd be willing to take on such a task weekly if he could guarantee the continued payoff, but we both know the seductive appeal would soon lose its luster.

My husband's toiling away on inefficient bureaucratic paperwork is an example of an act of service, one of the five "love languages" outlined in Dr. Gary Chapman's book of the same name. Love languages are ways in which we humans express care for one another. The five love languages are gifts (not necessarily expensive; they can be handwritten notes or thoughtful little trinkets), quality time (phones away, offering full attention), words of affirmation (*I love yous, thank you for . . . , I appreciate _____ about you*), acts of service (changing the oil in your car, cooking dinner), and physical touch (affection and sex).

Each of us has one or two primary love languages or ways in which we like to be shown love by our partners. Where we often miss the mark, though, is when we unconsciously employ our own preferred love language rather than theirs. So, for example, if my primary love language is gifts, I might spend a good amount of time choosing a thoughtful gift for my husband, only to find myself hurt and confused when I receive a lackluster thanks for what felt, to me, like a generous and obvious display of care. If I am aware, however, that his primary love language is time, I can set aside a few hours in our hectic schedules to turn off all devices and sit down together to play a game or just chat. In tending to him in his love language, he feels more connected, understood, and appreciated.

So, regardless of how devoted we are to our careers, we must be sure to turn some of that time, energy, and attention toward our partners as well. If we become complacent and disconnected, we are more apt to fall into that fruitless Janet Jackson what-have-you-done-for-me-lately mindset. The Partners Mindful Break is about flipping that unhelpful attitude on its head, inquiring of ourselves instead, "What have *I* done for *you* lately?"

Granted, if your relationship is of the newer, honeymoon-stage variety, this may not require a reminder, though this mindful break still applies. If your union has existed for a while, you know life can periodically get in the way. This mindful break need not require a romantic partnership. It can also be applied to colleagues, friends, or family members, as we all need some mutual support to keep our work–life balance in good working order. Though a simple concept, the five love languages is incredibly powerful and often life-changing when put to good use.

The Partners Mindful Break

I encourage you to share this break with your partner. Who wouldn't want to be asked how they like to be shown love? Not to mention that it will clue your partner in to *your* primary love language. Score!

1 First, identify your own main love language (or top two if it is impossible to choose just one).

2 Either by asking explicitly or making an educated guess (I recommend the former), consider which of the five is your partner's favorite.

3 Experiment with the various ways you can show your partner love in his language. Notice and savor the satisfaction this provides both him and you. Sit back and watch your relationship thrive.

4 When he makes an attempt to use your love language, acknowledge and thank him for his efforts.

5 Revisit this mindful break and your love languages periodically, as they can shift according to the various seasons of our lives. (Before kids, my primary would have been affection; now acts of service clearly tops my list.)

6 When applying this mindful break to friends or colleagues, make an educated guess, based on what you know of their personalities, to show your care and respect through the love language you imagine is best suited to them rather than automatically defaulting to using your own.

7 Have fun, be creative, and think outside the box. I have a feeling my husband will be on the lookout for other convoluted, laborious documents in need of his attention. Score again.

Hot in Here

⸻

A woman is like a tea bag—you can't tell how strong she is until you put her in hot water.

—Eleanor Roosevelt

The Hot in Here Mindful Break is all about cooling ourselves down whenever our internal temperature rises involuntarily—for all sorts of reasons. For example, we can find ourselves heating up from red-faced embarrassment after unwittingly inserting our foot in our mouth with a superior, as a result of self-induced pressure in the midst of a presentation, from the sweltering effects of an intraoffice thermostat set permanently too high, after a brisk 5-Minute Walk Mindful Break (page 95), or perhaps even after encountering the cute barista when grabbing our morning cup of joe.

Though this mindful break is useful for us all, regardless of age, it might especially speak to those at a more, shall we say, mature stage in our lives. Those of us in middle age once found it hard to imagine ever arriving here—and for many of you younger women, I'm sure you still do, but keep reading! I get it. That I am smack dab in the thick of it still bewilders and astonishes me on a regular basis. Don't get me wrong; aside from the expanding waistline, emerging bingo wings, and unpredictable mood swings, there is a lot to be said for this distinguished stage of our lives—a measure of hard-earned wisdom, accumulated career and life experience, and the increased capacity for mentoring. Yet, within this lovely phase of midlife womanhood, there nonetheless persists one of the most oft-lamented elements: *the battle of the dreaded hot flash.*

In case you have managed to remain blissfully unacquainted with the lurid details, hot flashes have been described as "typically triggered by falling estrogen levels during perimenopause . . . [and] often start with a sense of warmth, which can escalate to feelings of intense heat usually felt in the scalp, face and chest area. A flash may also be accompanied by tingling, nausea, increased heart rate, or perspiration."[14] Doesn't that sound like a treat?! Although each woman's journey through midlife is unique, according to statistics from Johns Hopkins Medicine, we women have a 75 percent chance of regularly encountering these inconvenient little adventures in temperature regulation at some point along the way.[15]

Among my girlfriends and me, hot flashes have become a notably hot (pun intended) topic of conversation. One of these beautiful women is so intimately familiar with them that she has learned to recognize an impending one about twenty seconds before it hits. This brief window enables her to at least (hastily, but appropriately) strip off some clothing, guzzle an ice-cold drink, or subtly commence fanning herself in an attempt to keep her internal temperature at more of a moderately sweltering rather than severely scorching point on the thermometer.

Believe it or not, there is an upside to all of this. Well, sort of; though we may not be in control over whether we are included in that 75 percent and cannot entirely eradicate these unpleasant little meltdowns, through decreasing our overall stress level we *can* learn to quell the magnitude of those erratic fiery hot flashes. The intensity and frequency of hot flashes can be ameliorated with stress-reduction practices.

The rising of our internal temperature, regardless of its origin and our age, can thankfully be refreshingly chilled as well. And that, my friend, is where the trusty Hot in Here Mindful Break comes to the rescue. Otherwise known as the cooling breath, this technique can be used anytime, anywhere. With practice, the amount of time we spend heated up can be shortened and lessened. Practice regularly so that when the unwanted internal fire begins, you are familiar, primed, and prepared.

The Hot in Here Mindful Break

❶ Sit or stand tall in a comfortable position and straighten the spine.

❷ Rather than resist the inevitable, relax your body and, as best you can, accept the arrival of the dear little hot flash, red face, or warmer climate, as struggling against it only tightens the muscles and worsens the symptoms.

❸ With the mouth open slightly, purse your lips as if ready to whistle.

❹ Inhaling slowly, feel the cool air move over the tongue and into the lungs.

❺ Allow the mouth to close and exhale slowly through the nose.

❻ Repeat as many times as needed.

Bedtime

S leepy + angry = *slangry*.
       My beloved family has coined this term to convey my slightly frightening mood when tiredness hits like a ton of bricks. After putting my six-year-old to bed, my husband, daughter, and I might sit down to take in a movie. Despite my best efforts to remain awake, sleepiness takes hold, and head bobbing ensues. This is when the exhaustion acquires a sense of urgency, and in a raspy, cranky voice, I proclaim that I must *immediately* get myself to bed. If one of them dares to suggest I muscle through ("Only fifteen more minutes until the end!"), my head spins around, eyes glowing crimson red, and *bam!*, I've arrived in the spine-chilling land of slangry. Everyone: *Watch out!* Fortunately, because I am aware of my limits and maintain a relatively routine schedule, this happens rarely. (Though my family might argue that a single occurrence is one too many.)

      If my slangry phenomenon resonates, you now have some proper nomenclature for your affliction (you're welcome). For some of us, bedtime has nothing to do with sleepiness and everything to do with increased anxiety and swirling thoughts, as bodies, perhaps slowing for the first time all day, and in seemingly futile fashion, await minds to follow. For others, bedtime is steadfastly postponed in spite of exhaustion and the nagging understanding that pushing those limits is not in our best interest.

So often we busy women sacrifice sleep in order to accomplish more or to attend just one more event (FOMO?), yet in reality this is counterproductive to our overall balance. Though the recommended number of nightly slumber hours for an adult is seven to nine, many of us expect to operate effectively on much less, voluntarily burning the candle at both ends in the name of work, productivity, or, we manage to convince ourselves, out of necessity. But sleep deprivation is no joke, wreaking havoc on our physical, mental, and emotional health. Sleeping less than seven hours a night negatively affects our reaction time as well as our ability to be productive and think creatively. As reported on the website Medical News Today, chronic insufficient sleep can lead to a weakened immune system, an increase in appetite and accompanying weight gain, heightened irritability, impaired ability to concentrate, and increased risk of depression and cardiovascular disease.[16] Wow, quite a list. Now you're certainly awake.

Granted, a sound night's sleep is not always under our control. Do your best to set up the conditions for a healthy seven to nine hours whenever possible. You can create a more soothing, restful drifting into dreamland by practicing the Bedtime Mindful Break.

The Bedtime Mindful Break

Feel free to use some or all of the tips from the menu below:

- Whenever possible, do not allow yourself to slip into slangry land. *Please*, when you start to feel sleepy, stop fighting it and go to bed!

- Keep a notebook by your bedside to jot down random thoughts, lists, or reminders that insist on your immediate attention. By transferring them from your brain to the page, your mind is off the hook and more able to settle.

- Write down three successes and three "gratitudes" for that day.

- Take a few deep breaths and stretch your body, taking care to keep the pace calm and sleep inducing rather than energizing.

- Maintain a work-free, screen-free, relaxing ambience and cool temperature in the bedroom. Keep alcohol and food consumption a few hours before bedtime to a minimum.

- Meditate for five minutes (see Meditation: It's Not What You Think, page 22).

- Practice a body scan lying down (see Desk Body Scan Mindful Break, page 50).

- Read an inspirational book or an upbeat work of fiction. This is not the ideal time for that page-turner. Find a story that will help lull you into a peaceful slumber.

- If insomnia persists, try the Wide-Awake Mindful Break, page 119, and repeat.

Wishing you deep, peaceful sleep, and the enduring absence of slangry-hood.

Wide-Awake
(aka 4-7-8 Breath)

I love my gynecologist. *Hmm,* that does not sound right. What I mean is, having received her attentive care over many years and through various stages of my adult life, I have grown quite fond of her. Her warm demeanor and familiarity render my obligatory annual appointment less unpleasant than it might otherwise be. During the past few visits, as I've moved squarely into middle age, she has begun inquiring into the quality of my sleep. "Any issues with insomnia?" she asks. I get the distinct impression she is just biding her time until it is my turn. Not that she wishes it upon me, of course, just that she seems most confident I will eventually answer in the affirmative, finding my place among all the other middle-aged women suffering from sleep maladies.

"Not if everyone lets me sleep," I answer. Which is true. If the teenager is not clattering around in the kitchen at 11:00 PM, if the six-year-old is not dreaming about monsters, if the dog does not need to go out before dawn, then, yes, I can sleep. Falling asleep is never the issue. When I am awakened and remain so for longer than four seconds, however, all bets are off. I will surely see the clock turn a few hours before slumber returns once again. Sometimes this stretch of sleeplessness is peaceful, my mind drifting along aimlessly in the silence of the night. Other times the mind-chatter game begins. Occasionally, the chatter picks up steam and takes on a life of its own, every tiny daytime worry magnified and sucked into the rapidly expanding sphere of anxiety and angst. Once I reach this point, no amount of reason can calm down the drama mama who has taken over my mind. This is when I pull out the Wide-Awake Mindful Break, otherwise known as the 4-7-8 breath, metaphorically leading the now frantic drama mama by the hand and eventually tucking her in to peaceful dreamland for the night. So if, despite your best efforts, insomnia insists on disturbing your precious peaceful slumber, this mindful break will offer you some middle-of-the-night relief.

The Wide-Awake Mindful Break

- First, take a moment to turn your attention to the body, relaxing any tight muscles as you briefly scan through each part.

- Gently place your tongue against the back of your upper teeth and allow it to remain there.

- Now slowly inhale through your nose as you silently count to four. Hold your breath for the count of seven and then exhale gently through your mouth to the count of eight. Repeat this cycle as many times as you'd like.

- Periodically check in with your body, continuing to soften any tense muscles.

- Note that the 4-7-8 breath is not the equivalent of a prescribed sleep aid, sending you effortlessly off to dreamland within a few short minutes, but a simple way to calm down the busy mind that may have revved up your body as well.

- Once you have quieted your mind and body, you may choose to read a good book or practice a body scan lying down (see Desk Body Scan Mindful Break, page 50).

- Remember, we cannot force sleep, as it will only result in frustration and further sleeplessness. Remind yourself that we are more resilient than we think and can operate reasonably well on much less sleep than is ideal. As best you can, set up the conditions so sleep can come to you. Sweet dreams, my friend.

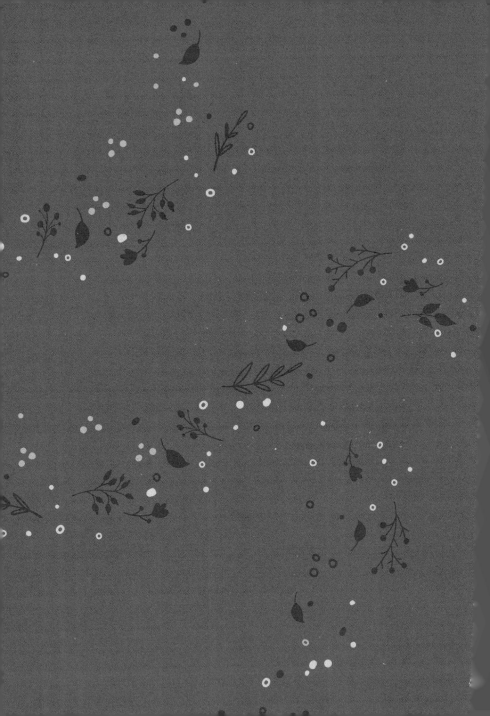

CHAPTER 2

Becoming Mindful Breaks

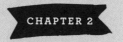

Once we have had the opportunity to usher in some calm with mindfulness, we are able to dream bigger and live more joyfully, with greater balance. But before all else we need to ensure we are not standing in our own way. We may have identified the most fulfilling, perfectly-suited-to-us goals, but without first addressing self-imposed barriers in the form of limiting beliefs and self-doubt, they will remain just that—unattained goals. Without bringing them into the light and flipping them on their heads, our growth and ability to achieve will always be stunted.

Enter the mighty Becoming Mindful Breaks. These are short practices designed to kindly highlight those areas preventing you from becoming your most awesome self—limiting beliefs, lack of confidence, and insufficient assertiveness—so you can move on to the action, the success, the achievements to which you aspire. The Becoming Mindful Breaks provide simple micro-action steps to ramp up your energy, bolster your confidence, and practice assertive communication. You will learn how to feel your best, work hard, play hard, and push yourself out of your comfort zone in fun, manageable ways. The Becoming Mindful Breaks offer up that extra mindfulness edge so that you can go out there and take on the world with authentic self-assurance and ease.

Do Not Fear Mistakes: There Are None

———

Great things happen when you don't know what you are doing.

—Dave Grohl

"Do not fear mistakes: There are none." Easy for me to say? Well, no, not really. Although one of my favorite personal mistakes ultimately led to the successful publishing of my first book, this Miles Davis quote, which is posted visibly in my office, is a reminder that there is always a valuable lesson in our perceived mistakes, even the wretchedly painful ones that in the moment appear cataclysmic and irreversible. This is not to say that we would never alter some of our decisions—given the retrospective opportunity. In reality, the best we can do is learn from our missteps, make amends if necessary, and usher our newfound knowledge into the present, allowing it to inform our future with wisdom.

The words we choose to describe our blunders matter. Our minds often transform a mere thought into a hard fact, often without our consent. A simple "mistake" can easily morph into a big fat FAILURE if we aren't cautious about how we perceive it. Which is why I have long bristled at the word *failure*, finding it too finite, too definite, and much too all-or-nothing in its formulation. And because I have repeatedly observed how "failure" paralyzes us in an unending cycle of fearing more of the same, I am opposed to even permitting it full-word status outside of mental quotation marks and often refer to it as "the other F-word." It is infinitely more productive, motivating, and sanity preserving to practice reframing the concepts of "mistakes" and "failures" as the potential learning opportunities they are.

When it comes to risking failure, each of us falls on the continuum from cripplingly risk averse to consummate adrenaline junkie—most of us not camped at the edge of either extreme but leaning clearly one way or the other. Ideally, we want to find ourselves in the center, making wise, deliberate decisions without allowing fear to immobilize us.

In my younger years, perfectionist tendencies and the fear of failure kept me playing it safe most of the time. As I have grown older, I have learned to nudge, and occasionally (lovingly) shove, myself more toward the center. As with learning any new skill, this was initially frightening, but it has become less so with practice. Despite my earlier risk aversion, I have nevertheless managed to experience my share of setbacks. It's just as important, if not more so, to discuss our losses than to underscore our wins. Success is decidedly not linear. Colin Jost of *Saturday Night Live* said it better than I ever could: "We have to remember that progress isn't just a straight line upward. . . . It's a weird roller coaster where sometimes you're screaming for joy and other times you're barfing in your own face." Pretty much.

Some time ago, having run my solo psychotherapy practice for a number of years, I was approached to join a local group practice. Enticed by the promise of a highly promoted mindfulness program and a decrease in administrative tasks, after much deliberation I was sold. The new position required that I also leave the well-established mindfulness organization in which I taught alongside people I respected and whose friendship I valued. Although it was not an easy decision, it seemed too good an opportunity to pass up. My leave-taking was not entirely well received, and some relationships were sorely damaged in the process.

The wheels were set in motion as I started the numerous tedious steps necessary to make the changeover. A few short weeks before the final transition, I began to have serious doubts about signing on with this new practice. I vividly recall returning home from a long bike ride, anxiety weighing heavily on my chest. Tentatively, I shared my fears with my husband, uncertain if what I was experiencing was typical fear or if it was my intuition desperately attempting to communicate more serious problems. With reassurances from my husband I forged full steam ahead, resigned at that point to having already signed on the dotted line. I pushed the trepidation down and replaced it with an enthusiastic, positive mindset for what I hoped was to come.

Predictably, it did not take long to recognize that my intuition had been correct; the new group was clearly not a good match. My client schedule was sparse at first, so I began using the open appointment slots to create blog posts, initially to promote the group's mindfulness program. I wrote about common themes my clients discussed, about my experiences as a mom to a then infant and preteen, and how mindfulness helped me maintain sanity. I continued writing and writing, the ideas flowing freely, until it dawned on me that I had compiled a book-length document. I began thinking about offering independent workshops while continuing to offer therapy and general mindfulness for the group practice. When I pitched my idea of independent workshops to the group owners they were not on board, making it clear that my offering any classes autonomously was out of the question. There was my answer. I could not, in good conscience or with any amount of self-respect, stay, even if I was not altogether prepared to leave. Back to square one, starting over with the countless tedious tasks of opening my own practice. Fear. No income. Change. Again.

Love your mistakes as much as your accomplishments. Because without mistakes, there wouldn't be any accomplishments.
—**Unknown**

Through it all I managed to survive and, after a few anxious months, began to thrive. I relocated to a beautiful, breathable, Zen-like space much closer to home. I righted the wrongs, repairing the broken relationships with those colleagues. I carried on writing, eventually signing with a literary agent and landing a book deal with a reputable publisher. That scary, seemingly enormous failure thrust me out of complacency, forcing me to make changes I would not otherwise have made, and it continues to this day to lead me in fascinating directions. Now, so much happier, I work autonomously, able to collaborate with whomever I choose, create my own schedule, follow my curiosity, and take on whichever projects light a fire within.

The Do Not Fear Mistakes: There Are None Mindful Break

❶ Designate where you fall on the risk-taking continuum: Do you tend to play it safe, hang back, and think long and hard about decisions? Do you often regret not having jumped in and experienced adventures, large or small? Or do you find yourself frequently regretting impulsive decisions? Are you regularly drawn to that addictive adrenaline rush from just going for it? Regardless of where you fall on the spectrum, reserve judgment about who you are or how you have behaved in the past. This is not about self-criticism but about kind awareness. Self-acceptance must first occur before we can create any mindful positive change.

If you tend to be risk averse, your next step is to work on stepping out of your comfort zone in tiny, manageable ways. Granted, we may not make as many missteps if we are always playing it safe, but we are also not living up to our full potential and end up stunting opportunities for growth.

If you are more of a natural risk taker, your objective is to stop and notice your body sensations before you leap, paying attention to what they may be communicating and honing your ability to notice and follow your intuition over time.

❷ If you are deliberating about whether to take a leap: Regardless of whether you are risk averse or risk adoring, first get quiet in order to listen to your body, as it provides valuable information. You must physically stop to do this. Briefly scan through the body from head to toe, staying curious about any sensations and making mental notes of what you observe.

If it is difficult to notice any sensations at all, do not be discouraged. Each time you practice this mindful break, you increase your familiarity with your own unique body sensations, becoming more in tune with what is normal—and what is not—for you. Typically, we experience sensations tied to emotions somewhere between the head and the stomach or lower back. For example, you might feel muscle tension in your head, neck, or back. Perhaps it feels as if an elephant has taken a seat atop your chest or butterflies are trapped in your stomach. These unpleasant sensations commonly signal an unhealthy, unwise choice. Conversely, ask yourself if there is a general sense of ease, calm, and relaxed muscles. This usually means you are proceeding in the right direction.

Even if you are skilled at noticing sensations, it isn't always clear what they represent. Or, as in my case, we recognize the sensations but doubt the message out of fear, avoidance, or denial. Since we know that attempting something new often also entails some level of fear, our goal is to distinguish between natural trepidation (take the risk) and our intuition screaming *NO!* (consider turning back). This, too, requires practice and never entirely becomes foolproof. Provided we gather facts and heed our intuition, we can be assured that we have done our best in that moment, whether we succeed immediately or not.

(Note: It is useful to practice noticing body sensations on a regular basis, not just when facing a difficult choice. Practicing only "crisis meditation" can be helpful, but isn't ideal. See the Desk Body Scan, page 50.)

❸ **If you are recovering from a "mistake":** Take a deep breath and offer yourself compassion for the suffering (see Kindness Mindful Break, page 55, for more on self-compassion). Remind yourself that you are not alone; everyone has a similar story to share. I know this may be irritating to hear right now, but it will ring true later. Regardless of whether you did not notice informative body sensations, interpreted them wrong, or chose not to heed them, there is always a lesson to be learned—even if it is not immediately clear. Sometimes the best you can do is breathe, put one foot in front of the other, refuse to let fear keep you down, and use what you've learned to wisely, kindly inform your next decision.

The Magic Wand

*The world only exists in your eyes—your conception of it.
You can make it as big or as small as you want to.*

—F. Scott Fitzgerald

Play along for a moment: Imagine I possess a powerful magic wand, able to grant you a wish for one particular talent or ability that has, until this point in time, been elusive. What would you choose? (No, you are not allowed to wish for more wishes. Play nice.) Your granted ability can be realistic or outlandish, work related or personal. This is an opportunity to dream a little, setting all practical logistics aside.

You may have always wished you could carry a tune, fantasizing about touring the world with your all-female punk-rock band. Maybe you yearn for the ability to allow constructive feedback to roll easily off your back, instead of taking up a monthlong obsessive residence in your mind. Perhaps, like me, you aspire to be an effortless public speaker, bounding onto the stage with supreme confidence and ease, gazing out into a crowd of thousands, secure in the knowledge that your message will be articulately and perfectly delivered, exactly in tune with what the audience needs to hear.

It's OK if your wished-for ability is more superhero than practical, as the skills it grants are illuminating. These wishes help us recognize what we would like to modify about ourselves or our circumstances. It is then up to us to do the work to identify which pieces are under our control and the small, simple steps needed to get there.

For example, if you would love to possess X-ray vision, this desired ability might really be about wishing you could effectively read others' body language and tone in order to better understand them. (It's a good thing some wishes are not grantable in real life, as I imagine, in this case, you might arrive at work and quickly experience X-ray vision buyer's remorse. You may choose another wish. I am an understanding and benevolent magic wand wielder, after all.)

Let's say you choose the ability to fly. What about it is so appealing? The unencumbered freedom and weightlessness? The utter silence of the clouds? The bird's-eye view so distant from the stressors of daily life? A sense of ease? Excitement? Your answers are full of information. Right there is the good stuff. Where in your life can you obtain more of those qualities? If it is freedom and weightlessness you are after, try something completely out of your comfort zone, like zip-lining or skydiving. If it is a small dose of excitement you crave, perhaps embark on an adventurous daylong road trip to a destination you've never before visited. If it is ease and quiet you desire, sign up for a gentle yoga class or head to the woods for a peaceful nature walk.

As far as my desire to be an effortless public speaker, I'm still working on it. Over the course of many years I have pushed myself to be comfortable speaking to increasingly larger audiences, implementing the steps in this mindful break. In the future, when you catch me hanging with Oprah or tune in to my brilliant interview with Terry Gross, know that I'll be offering myself some serious high fives for my diligent hard work and the enchanting Magic Wand Mindful Break.

The Magic Wand Mindful Break

Have a pencil and paper handy to jot down some thoughts. This is for your eyes only, so no need for neatness or even total clarity. Keep it in positive terms, writing as if you have already received your superpower.

1 Take a few deep breaths and relax your body. Now think of an ability you wish you had. Imagine it being granted. Close your eyes and picture yourself completely embodying this skill. Notice what about it is so appealing. What aspects of this wish resonate with you? Jot down some ideas. For example: *As a powerful public speaker, I am completely at ease in front of a massive audience or on live national television, totally self-assured that my message resonates with the crowd and that it offers a clear, valuable lesson.*

2 Next, start with the wish and move backward. Write down the actual steps it would take to get there. How much of it is under your control? Before you answer in the negative, pause and reconsider. We often have more choice than we realize at first glance, even if in small ways. It's helpful to think in future tense to envision the steps." For example, *I will offer talks to large audiences, and before that, in small venues. I will also be featured on prerecorded and live local TV shows.*

❸ Break down those steps even further. *I will design and practice my signature talk in front of a mirror and small audience. I will videotape myself in order to hone my presentation and delivery. I will reach out to colleagues and related contacts about offering my talk in various settings.*

❹ Identify one micro-step to start with today. Write that down. *E-mail my friend today to let her know I will be sending her an outline of my talk by next Friday. Ask her to keep me accountable by following up.* Notice the shift into present tense. Getting started is often the most challenging part of the process. Don't think too many steps ahead, prompting overwhelm and paralysis. One single completed micro-step builds on another until, one day, you will look back in wonder at how far you've come in developing your magic power.

❺ Revisit this mindful break periodically to congratulate yourself for the micro-steps you have completed or continue to work on. Determine what your next small steps will be and what needs to be modified. There are always ways to improve, grow, and continue nudging ourselves out of our comfort zones. Keep developing; keep pushing, just don't forget to congratulate yourself for your effort and progress along the way.

Body Love

Body love. An oxymoron, you say? For most of us, it certainly is.

Have you seen the hit show *The Marvelous Mrs. Maisel*? Set in the 1950s, the show portrays just how much attention and pressure was put on women to always appear slender and put-together. In one scene, the lead character, Midge Maisel, newly married, goes to bed for the night with full makeup and perfectly styled hair, waits patiently until her new husband falls blissfully asleep, then hops out of bed to wash it all off, only to make sure she gets up in the morning well before her hubby so she can guarantee looking perfectly presentable for him once again. Can you imagine? Another scene finds Midge meticulously measuring the circumference of her thigh, then painstakingly recording it in her daily log.

As absurd as this scene first appears, have we really come that far? Sure, the media has slowly begun shifting toward body positivity and maintaining a healthy weight; nevertheless, there remains strong pressure to be thin, fit, and young.

In Your Inner Bully Mindful Break (see page 140), I share my own perfectionistic body image struggles throughout my teens and early twenties. In hindsight, I am horrified at how much time, energy, and brainpower I spent worrying about what I did or did not eat and how I appeared to others. I had bought in to society's pervasive message that, as a developing woman, I should not take up too much space in the world.

Thankfully, in my twenties, I learned to exercise, eat moderately, and judge myself less. As I grew to respect and care for myself more, my weight seemed to take care of itself. It's not that I never gave it a thought but, for the most part, it became a nonissue.

Enter my late forties. My typically robust metabolism began to slow; my body grew softer in new and different areas. Once my fiftieth birthday hit, in the midst of a pandemic, all bets were off. I looked in the mirror one day, shocked to see the body of my mother at middle age staring back at me. What happened to that thirty-year-old body I still imagine I inhabit?

In all my years of working with women, I have yet to meet one who *loves her body*. I mean really, truly loves it and would not change a thing, given the chance. The extent to which each of us focuses on our body image ranges anywhere from "What body?" to near-constant obsession. Wherever we fall on the continuum, we can all spend more time appreciating our beautiful bodies—regardless of size or shape—and mining sensations for all sorts of valuable information.

The Body Love Mindful Break

Beware the judging. Start by paying attention to when you are negatively critiquing your body, simply name it *judging*, and offer yourself a bit of compassion for this unhelpful habit.

Name what you appreciate. We know that positive reinforcement is motivating, yet so many of us are downright cruel to ourselves when it comes to our bodies. By intentionally appreciating all that our bodies do for us, we promote a healthier relationship with our own strong, imperfect bods. Notice how it serves you well, how it functions automatically, how strong it is, how miraculous. For example, *I have strong legs that allow me to walk miles at a time. This body birthed two healthy children. These broad shoulders carry and support countless responsibilities.*

Create body love notes. *I am strong. I am healthy. My body is beautiful as it is.* I don't care if it feels cheesy; it works. Write them on sticky notes and place them where you will see them. Put a reminder on your phone to tell yourself each day. Make it a daily habit.

Recognize sensations. Deliberately tune into body sensations as invaluable sources of information. There are a number of ways to do this—with a brief body scan, yoga, stretching, or any form of mindful movement. How does your body feel after a good night's sleep, eating a healthy meal slowly, walking briskly in the sunshine, or a three-breath hug? Pleasant sensations point to what we might cultivate more of. Unpleasant sensations signal unwise decisions, unhealthy relationships, and unproductive situations. When we investigate our body sensations, we find infinite amounts of useful information. The more we practice noticing, the more we become tuned in to subtle clues.

Step outside yourself. Think about the women in your life. What do you appreciate about their bodies? Rather than comparing them to your own self-image, consider their beautiful, varied shapes and sizes. Kindly and firmly apply some of that positive regard to yourself.

This powerful combination of intentionally appreciating and tuning in to sensations will not only help you regard your body with a little more tenderness but offer you valuable wisdom as well. It's time for you to start offering your gorgeous, strong bod some love.

Your Inner Bully

Every cell in your body is eavesdropping on your thoughts.
—Deepak Chopra

My inner critic is a biatch. A powerful word, I concur, but it is fitting, I assure you. As a perfectionistic teen, my inner critic was a downright bully: a near-constant companion, laser-focused on my appearance and hypercritical of any perceived bodily defect, particularly consumed with the number on the bathroom scale that never seemed to dip low enough. Her persistent influence convinced me to expend entirely too much time dieting and self-critiquing my (*gasp!*) slender 115-pound youthful body. She also demanded I earn near-perfect grades, be a people pleaser despite any detriment to myself, and smile—always smile.

My inner bully was constantly busy hurling negative feedback my way, and she would not be caught dead offering up an ounce of praise or positive reinforcement. Her role was to keep a vigilant eye on me and a running tally of what needed improvement or was deemed, according to her strict assessment, to be lacking. I suppose for a time she kept me on my toes, ensuring that life ran smoothly and satisfactorily, but this constant barrage of negativity always comes at an eventual cost. An inwardly overwhelmed high school junior, I appeared, ostensibly, to be at the top of my game. In the middle of a quiet study hall, however, I experienced what turned out to be my first (and thankfully only, to this date) panic attack, though it took years for me to recognize it as one. It took another few years before I managed to let go of some of the perfectionism, allowing my inner bully to *chill out*, at least a bit.

As I made my way into my early twenties and began coming into my own, I also learned not to take my harshly belittling inner bully so seriously. I even went so far as to personify her, attributing fictional human characteristics to this previously dreaded force, eventually landing on the name *Marge*. In my twisted imagination, Marge resembled her garish Simpson namesake, all lavender bouffant, tightly fitting clothes, and tawdry makeup. My Marge deviated from the infamous Simpson in that her deeply furrowed brow was bookended between two squinted eyes, exposing her perennially irritated and disapproving disposition. My Marge did not instill confidence, a sense of worthiness, or appreciation for my quirky quirks. Oh no; she made it her *job* to tear me down and seemed to enjoy it, no less.

Human nature is such that we all have an active internal dialogue, often an inner bully of sorts (some of us have a crowd of them) who veers firmly toward the negative unless we train her otherwise. Her power runs the gamut from an excessively influential figure to one who makes only a rare cameo. Within our inner bully's commentary, we may recognize an overcritical parent or trusted adult from childhood. Perhaps we find she was born out of societal pressure and expectations of what we were told a woman should be. Perhaps she is some combination of the two.

Whatever the case, it's important to recognize that your inner bully's mere existence is not at all a problem. We all have some version of her lurking around. The question is how we perceive and respond to her. Treating our inner bully much like we might approach the classroom variety, when we recognize and call out the unacceptable oppressive behavior, we disempower both the harsh message and the bully herself.

It has taken plenty of time and patience on my part, but my Marge doesn't deem it worthwhile to make an appearance as often as she once did—save for when I am royally exhausted, emotionally depleted, or in the throes of an especially challenging case of PMS. *Then* she seems to be crouching in the shadows, ready to pounce on my mostly dormant insecurities and self-doubt. *You're going to wear that?* she asks, a singular eyebrow raised in disdain. *Hmm, interesting choice. You said what to your colleague? Wow, OK,* she chides, judgment oozing out of every makeup-caked pore.

With a good deal of practice on my part in using the steps below, Marge has lost much of her power over me. Now when she shows up, I am able to greet her with a bit of kindness. *Oh, hey, Marge,* I say with a casual wave of the hand. *What's up?* Because, though Marge can still act like a bit of a biatch, she has also grown paradoxically kind of sweet, in my estimation. As much as she can act the part of the quintessential mean girl, I have also come to feel some compassion for her—for her misguided attention to unimportant, impossible standards; for all the time and energy unnecessarily spent on futile striving.

And if she arrives at a moment when I'm feeling especially emotionally evolved and altruistic, I might even thank her for her well-meaning efforts, for her robust fondness for setting me on the "right" path, however ill advised. Marge desperately wants me to be the best I can be, after all. When we dive deeper still, she only hopes to protect me from any potential hurtful critique from the outside world. If my tale of Marge is even remotely recognizable to you, get to work on this mindful break.

Your Inner Bully Mindful Break

❶ First, assess your own inner bully. Are you already familiar with her? While some of us feel as if ours is virtually a conjoined twin, others have never paused to notice her existence. Congratulate yourself for noticing, as it is in the power of awareness that positive change can occur.

❷ Grant that inner bully a suitable name. What fits? Voldemortica? Helga? Mrs. Hassenpfeffer? Feel free to borrow *Marge*, if you'd like. I don't think she'd mind.

❸ Don't resist your inner bully or attempt to banish her to the land of misfits. In fact, *I invite you to invite her* to take a seat right alongside you. She is more than welcome to hang out and incessantly chatter away in your ear as long as she'd like. You are not required to heed her advice. Allow that chatter to fall to the background, much like unpleasant elevator Muzak. You know full well that it's there, but it isn't at the forefront of your attention.

❹ Although she might act like a complete biatch, remember that your inner bully is still a part of you, albeit one whose opinion you should disregard. Attempt to offer her some compassion for her misguided attempts, perhaps even thanking her for her concern. If you feel resistant to this suggestion, no need to judge yourself. Gently try it repeatedly, without forcing. This often takes time and practice.

❺ Offer yourself (this time all of you, not just the inner-bully part) kindness for the challenge and sometimes suffering we encounter with this antagonistic character. Place your hands over your heart. Talk graciously to yourself, as you would to a loved one or best friend.

❻ We need to not only keep our inner bully in her proper place but also counterbalance her negativity with credit for what we do well. (See the High Fives Mindful Break, page 183, and Your Inner Mentor, page 145, to positively reinforce all that is awesome about you.)

Your Inner Mentor

The way to develop the best that is in a person is by appreciation and encouragement.

—Charles Schwab

Recently diagnosed with a particular form of chronic lung disease, Monica came to see me after a frightening health episode related to her illness. The forty-seven-year-old stay-at-home mother of two school-age children leads an active life volunteering, exercising, and taxiing her kids to various events. As a healthy nonsmoker, the pronouncement came as a shock. The diagnosis fresh, Monica was still researching and digesting its life-changing ramifications. We began focusing on her panic and worried thoughts, specifically the unfathomable fear of dying and leaving her two children behind. Learning some calming mindful breaks, such as Wide-Awake, page 119, and the Triangle Tune-In, page 45, enabled Monica to better ride out those scary thought waves without being completely pulled under.

Intelligent and insightful, Monica was also interested in exploring what wisdom might be gleaned from this recent health struggle. Explaining that she had typically "played it safe" in her life, opting for comfort and security over adventure and adrenaline, Monica then went on to share a story that she had carried in her memory for decades.

As a young teen, Monica loved to act onstage in school productions but was insecure about her inexperience with dancing. One day, her beloved drama teacher, Mrs. H., encouraged her to give it a shot. Mrs. H. was a warm, boisterous, red-haired spitfire who could be quite convincing. Solely due to Mrs. H.'s urging, Monica relented and purchased her first and only pair of tap shoes, and she repeatedly rehearsed the dance number. She was especially nervous up on the school's old wooden auditorium stage, as its years of wax and wear rendered it slippery, particularly in those unfamiliar tap shoes. On the day of the dress rehearsal, wholly out of her element, Monica traipsed up on that stage and tapped—with slight, carefully controlled, cautious movements. Watching intently from the wings, Mrs. H. bellowed an earnest plea: "Dance, Monica, dance!" Monica got out of her head, let go of her inhibited tapping and, feeling daring and free, she danced her little teenage heart out.

That, Monica said, is exactly how she intends to live her life now—by heeding Mrs. H.'s assertion to "dance, Monica, dance!" Monica has promised herself to take up more space in the world, to go out and taste life, to stop playing it so damn safe. Mrs. H., a true mentor in every sense, not only offered Monica permission to release her self-consciousness and *dance with her whole being* but implored her to do so as if her life depended on it.

We all have a Mrs. H. living inside of us: an inner mentor, a wise adviser to compassionately guide and cheer us on—if we take the time to invite and access her. Your inner mentor can be in the flesh or fictitious. She is that wise woman (or man) you might be fortunate enough to have encountered in real life or the one you wish you had. She is a piece of you, albeit a part we often dismiss or ignore if we even recognize her presence at all. This mindful break is all about the ability to access our inner wisdom without getting in our own way—offering ourselves permission to desire, to speak up, to dance. Monica found her own inner mentor in the form of Mrs. H. Are you ready to search for yours?

Your Inner Mentor Mindful Break

Imagine your inner mentor and bring her to life in your mind. Do this with a light attitude, as an experiment in curiosity and exploration. If this is difficult at first, know that it might require a bit of practice before you can comfortably conjure her up. If you are fortunate enough to have your own real-life Mrs. H., recall her facial features, expressions, the sound of her voice, your memory of her in as much detail as possible. If she is of your own creation, allow her to become just as real. Picture her face, her hair, her smile. What is she wearing? How does she carry herself? Imagine the expression on her face when she looks at you. Whether real or imagined, allow her imperfections.

The most important qualifications are that she adores you, believes in you, is benevolent, and that you trust her.

Imagine her sitting across from you with a cup of tea. What is it she wants you to know? How does she advise you about who you are, the direction your life is headed, and what she wishes for you? How does it feel to hear these things? What resonates?

As you continue this experiment, becoming more familiar with your inner mentor, you can present her with your most burning questions. What would you like to ask? How does she answer? Ultimately, of course, she is you and your wisdom. Let her offer you that well-deserved comfort, compassion, and guidance.

Communication

*Everyone is interesting. If you're ever bored in a
conversation, the problem's with you, not the other person.*
—Matt Mullen

Bring to mind a time when you felt completely heard, seen, and
validated by someone. This needn't be a perfect moment, but
rather one that conveyed a sincere attempt at full attention and
understanding. You may even tear up at the thought, as it is such
a rare occurrence for most of us. So rare, in fact, that some of us
struggle to conjure up a single memory of one at all. (Go to the
Play Hooky Mindful Break to read about my reaction to a connected moment, page 235.)

We've all endured conversations with others who are distracted and disengaged, and we walk away feeling minimized,
invalidated, perhaps even disrespected. Granted, it can be challenging to slow down and offer someone our undivided attention
in the middle of a busy, constantly connected world. Countless
devices, tasks, and people compete for our limited attention. It
can feel almost painful to rip ourselves away from the computer

screen when a colleague unassumingly interrupts our flow. When shifting gears while writing, it feels to me as if I am wrenching myself from another universe, reentering my body and the world of other living beings, and it requires a few seconds to effectively reintegrate.

That is on a typical day. When we are overwhelmed and under stress, however, the part of our brain in charge of executive function (responsible for paying attention and thinking flexibly) is inhibited, which means attention wanders and we are naturally not as receptive. When I am feeling time starved and rushed, I want desperately for my family to communicate quickly and efficiently, a reaction of which I am not proud. This is my cue to pause and recognize the restlessness, tense muscles, and urge to hop up and move. It is an indication to take a few deep breaths, relax those muscles, and remind myself how important this person is to me. It is a firm and kind suggestion for the frantic get-'er-done mode to slow down. Seldom an instantaneous shift, it usually requires a few go-rounds. I am certainly a work in progress.

This is mindful communication in action—the practice of bringing our full attention, with acceptance and without judgment, to the interaction at hand. When we breathe deeply, relax our muscles, and return to the present moment (exactly what we practice during meditation) we are able to engage in more open-minded communication. Being human, we all crave being heard, seen, and validated, whether we're conscious of it or not. It is not only a gift for the other person but we, as the tuned-in listener, benefit as well through an increased sense of connection.

Mindful communication enhances successful leadership and is a vital component for a more productive, innovative, and authentic work culture. Practicing it also boosts what researchers term *relational energy,* "the energy you get when you interact with someone who energizes you."[17] According to research at the University of Michigan's Ross School of Business, relational energy "turns out to be a big predictor of job performance and personal well-being. The more relational energy a leader exudes the better employees on that team perform in terms of productivity, absenteeism, engagement, and job retention."[18] That isn't to say you need to be charming or extroverted to succeed; on the contrary, relational energy is all about how others are left feeling after you interact with them.

Bring to mind a person with whom you've experienced relational energy, a person who is authentically positive and whose energy is contagious. It goes without saying that we want to surround ourselves with such people as much as possible—and most likely we intuitively do this already. More important and exciting is that we can learn to raise our own relational energy through the practice of mindful communication. Maya Angelou sums it up: "I've learned that people will forget what you said, people will forget what you did, but people will never forget how you made them feel." Yes, let us bestow more of that good energy.

The Communication Mindful Break

While interacting with another person, practice mindful communication. Ideally, practice it together.

❶ Deliberately allow a bit of silence to enter the conversation and take a few deep breaths. If the other person is not privy to your practice, you can do this subtly in your own mind. Make eye contact and relax your muscles. Remember that this calms the fight-or-flight reaction and allows you to access your wisdom, patience, and open-mindedness.

❷ Open to what is here. Accept the moment, the conversation, and the other person as nonjudgmentally as possible. When judgments do arise, notice them, and, as best you can, return your attention to the dialogue.

❸ Listen deeply, with plenty of space and time. Zip it! Let go of assumptions and that brilliant piece of wisdom you are desperate to share. With genuine curiosity, attempt to understand what they are conveying, perhaps imagining what it is like to be in their place.

❹ If your attention drifts off, simply take another breath and redirect your focus to the conversation.

❺ Speak the truth with kindness, relying on authenticity. Stop yourself from rehearsing how you anticipate the conversation will proceed—though for crucial, difficult conversations some forethought is fine and even recommended.

It is normal to cycle through these steps as needed throughout a single conversation. With attention to where you can improve in the future, be sure to applaud your efforts.

Unmute Yourself

You will be a revolutionary because any woman who is being authentic in her work will bring forth ideas and ways of working that run counter to the status quo of her company, industry, community—a status quo defined by masculine values and masculine ways of working.

—Tara Mohr

Beth, a midlevel manager in a national organization, spends most of her day interacting with colleagues through video chats and conference calls. She has always been apprehensive about public speaking and speaking up, especially on calls that include higher-ranking employees or a large number of participants. Despite the insightful comments that dwelled on the tip of her tongue during calls, Beth continued to mute both her computer and herself because she feared sounding unintelligent and possessing inadequate knowledge.

For years, Beth erroneously believed that her strong work ethic and accomplishments would speak for themselves and be sufficient to get her noticed by the higher-ups. As her career stagnated, though, she began to feel frustrated with the company and herself. Witnessing her struggle, a trusted female leader advised Beth to "get comfortable with being uncomfortable." Following her leader's guidance, Beth resolved that in order to advance in her organization, she must unmute herself. Literally. "Now I'm off mute almost all the time asking questions and providing feedback (although at times I still do get nervous!). Ever since I unmuted myself, my career has taken off and so many new doors have been opened," she told me.

> *Connection is the energy that is created between people when they feel seen, heard and valued—when they can give and receive without judgment.*
> —Brené Brown

We women, especially, are muted in numerous ways: We're bulldozed over in conversation; we acquiesce, allowing someone else to take the floor out of deference; and, as in Beth's case, we sometimes choose to mute ourselves deliberately when questioning our knowledge or caving to insecurity. The poignant image of bravely pressing that unmute button reminds us to unearth our assertive voice, get comfortable with being uncomfortable, speak our wise truth, and contribute our unique, valuable input to the world.

The Unmute Yourself Mindful Break

❶ Identify the ways in which you literally or figuratively mute yourself. If you are already aware of this tendency, you know on which specific areas to focus. If not, you are

(a) the rare woman who naturally asserts herself easily and often, (b) like Beth, have worked diligently on your own version of this mindful break, or (c) not yet tuned in to it. To uncover more about option (c), think of a time when you suppressed a meaningful contribution to a conversation out of uncertainty. Do you allow others to take charge of interactions and meetings while you hang back and observe? If yes, you have been muted. Welcome to the club.

❷ Rather than self-judge, congratulate yourself for recognizing it, attending to it, and endeavoring to overcome it.

❸ As you prepare to unmute, recognize where you experience the inevitable discomfort in your body. Pounding heart? Sweaty 'pits? Shortness of breath? The unpleasantness in unmuting ourselves is real, palpable, and completely normal. Speak up in spite of it. In fact, know that the adrenaline generating those physical sensations can actually *enhance* your thinking and ability to articulate.

❹ Unmuting ourselves grows easier the more often we practice it—and eventually becomes freeing, empowering, and advantageous for all who benefit from your previously withheld wisdom and opinions.

❺ Take a deep breath, then go ahead and unmute yourself. Speak up. Make your point. Offer your feedback. Provide your opinion. It's time. You've got this.

Proof of Your Awesomeness

Promise me you'll always remember—you're braver than you believe, and stronger than you seem, and smarter than you think.
—Christopher Robin, from the Disney film *Pooh's Grand Aventure*

I have known plenty of smart, resourceful, and resilient women who, when considering a new career venture, staunchly doubt their obvious (to everyone else) capabilities. First is Carrie, a thirtysomething Ivy League MBA grad who introduced herself to me after I had given a talk on mindful motherhood some years back. She, about to launch a part-time coaching business (after staying home with her three children for a handful of years) and I, just venturing out with various new mindfulness workshops, quickly hit it off and began meeting up biweekly to discuss how to balance career goals with young children and countless other responsibilities. Carrie had read no less than forty books on launching a side hustle and, month after month, offered up pointed questions and observations about my work and aspirations. Yet here she was, seated across from me in our cozy café meeting spot, earnestly questioning the necessity of an expensive, time-consuming coaching certification program before comfortably offering up her talents to the world. She questioned not only her intellect but her ability to fit her vision of playing big into her full life.

Next is Greta, a recent college grad with a marketing and business degree whom I have worked with periodically for a decade. Mature, wise, and strong, Greta is also clear about her dream of operating her own full-time marketing business . . . eventually. After weighing the possibilities and discussing it with trusted advisers (who were divided in their opinions), she landed on the presumption that she first required more experience.

Greta, with more than a hint of resignation, opted for a lackluster, though secure, position within a small company. While I fully understand and respect her caution and diligence, I also have complete confidence that she is already more than adequately equipped to go at it on her own. I have no doubt one day she will.

What Carrie and Greta have in common is a hefty dose of self-doubt along with an unfounded conviction that they are not yet ready—just one more training, class, certification, or [fill in the blank]—to dive into the career they are not only highly qualified for but clearly well suited to. They doubted themselves and their ability to create balance in their lives along the way.

When embarking on a challenge outside of our comfort zone, it is normal and expected that many thoughts will arise as to why we aren't ready—even more so in women than in men (see Why Not Me?, page 174). In a well-known review of human resource records at Hewlett-Packard, Katty Kay, BBC news anchor, reported that when applying for a promotion, women only pursued the opportunity if they considered themselves to have met 100 percent of the position qualifications, whereas the men felt comfortable throwing their hat in the ring when they believed they could fulfill 60 percent.[19] Self-doubt, fear, and worry are all unconscious self-protective measures, though often misguided and overzealous. Which is precisely why we women, especially, need to be vigilant about our appearance and accuracy. Otherwise, lack of self-assurance about our skills and capabilities can significantly hinder our growth and ability to take wise risks.

Kay goes on to say confidence is crucial because it "is a belief in one's ability to succeed, a belief that stimulates action. In turn, taking action bolsters one's belief in one's ability to succeed. So confidence accumulates—through hard work, through success, and even through failure." The Proof of Your Awesomeness Mindful Break is all about shoring up your confidence by diving into past accomplishments for evidence that you have what it takes to succeed and recalibrate balance, which you can then utilize when your self-confidence wanes. (For evidence of your grit and strengths, see also What Are Your Superpowers?, page 187.)

The Proof of Your Awesomeness Mindful Break

This break is most effective when written. Go grab a pen and notebook.

Identify a time when you succeeded at something—no need for an Olympic medal or Nobel Prize—any accomplishment you feel pride in will do. Maybe you conscientiously completed a project that originally felt daunting. Perhaps, as a mom, you handled a challenging childhood phase well. Maybe you saved up over a number of years to buy your first home.

If judgmental thoughts arise about what has not gone well or what you have not yet achieved, notice them and gently brush them aside. We are not interested in their negative chatter right now. Return as many times as necessary to the positives.

Now, with lavish, uninhibited praise, as if pumping yourself up with an enthusiastic pep talk, write about this accomplishment. (*You worked persistently and diligently, day after day, on your presentation*, etc.). As you revisit this success, recall moments of doubt or overwhelm that emerged in the process. How did you cope with or conquer them? What skills and attributes were required to make this happen? Let this sink in.

Write (addressing yourself) a brief reminder about how this is proof you are capable of reaching other dreams. *In spite of those doubts and great fear of speaking in front of your superiors, you worked your tail off to compile a compelling presentation. You dug down for some courage, took some deep breaths, got up in front of the entire staff, and rocked it. When you were finished, you were so proud and elated. This is proof that you are more than capable of handling whatever challenge comes your way.*

If you do not immediately feel fully convinced, no worries; just keep reminding yourself of what you have already accomplished as you put one foot in front of the other on the way to your dreams.

Best Possible Self

—

Dreams come true; without that possibility, nature would not incite us to have them.

—John Updike

While waiting to build my caseload after joining a group psychotherapy practice, I casually began writing informative blog posts about meditation and mindful breaks as an antidote to the busy, stressed-out state of motherhood many of my clients were experiencing. After a few months, it occurred to me that I had unwittingly compiled the potential beginnings of a full-length book. I considered self-publishing, but I opted to first pursue representation by a literary agent and the traditional publishing house route. The worst that could happen, I figured, was the accumulation of a slightly disheartening pile of rejection letters. (This book writing business comes up a lot—I believe for good reason—as it has been a huge accomplishment for me, one I have poured my heart and soul into. Indulge me, if you will.)

Around the same time, and prior to reaching out to any agents, I enrolled in the Greater Good's Science of Happiness online continuing education course. One early morning, following a homework writing prompt, I sat to scrawl, stream-of-consciousness-like, for twenty minutes about my ideal life in the future. I imagined it as a movie in which everything had gone as well as possible, having achieved all of my dreams and goals. The following is an excerpt of what emerged on the page:

I am so thrilled that I have landed a wonderful agent who is energetic and believes in my book. Because of her, I have finalized a book deal with a publisher! I can't believe this is happening. The book is finished and now just coming back for last-minute edits. I remember last year at this time—how the doubt would arise— should I even finish this book? *Something told me to just keep going with it. It feels like all of my hard work is paying off.*

I allowed myself to dream, wrote specifically *as if it had already happened*, and voilà (well, with a reasonable amount of time, energy, and wise guidance by a trusted mentor), I secured that agent, signing on the dotted line with a fantastic New York publisher. Not only that, but this intentionally crafted labor of love, *Breathe, Mama, Breathe*, is a hit with mamas all over the world, and my second book (the one in your hands) has lovingly been birthed as well.

That original writing prompt was part of a research study showing evidence of how powerful setting specific, intentional goals can be.[30] This book is proof that when we picture ourselves living our dream, break the goal down into manageable steps, and are diligent and tenacious, accomplishments we may never have imagined possible become possible, indeed.

Take the time to write about your best possible self. Set aside those self-imposed limitations and doubts. Dream big, invite what arises, and play it out in detail. Then, start small and start now. You just might find yourself, a year from now, living the dream.

It's not so much that if we picture something happening, it certainly will happen (it's not magic) as that if we can't picture something happening, it probably won't. Envision the outcome you want.

—Martha Beck

The Best Possible Self Mindful Break

1 This mindful break is useful when done in your dazzling imagination but is definitely more powerful when written. Grab a pen and paper.

2 Imagine yourself in the future, your life going as well as you can possibly imagine. Write out a scene of your best possible self as if you were living it—the setting, conditions, and your overall state of mind. Where are you living? With whom? How do you spend your time? What lights you up?

What goals have you attained? What wishes have been ful-filled? How are you feeling—emotionally, mentally, phys-ically, and spiritually? Look around and tune in to your senses. What do you hear? Smell? Taste? Feel?

3 As you write stream-of-consciousness, set your self-imposed limitations and doubts aside. Keep it positive, dream big, and see what arises. The more detailed and descriptive you are, the better. In order to make our dreams a reality, we first need to know which direction we are headed.

4 Suppose I could guarantee the achievement of that dream if you begin with one small action toward it *today*. What will that be? Write it down and determine exactly when you will make that happen. Go out there, one step at a time, and turn those fictional dreams into reality.

Ego States

It is easier to act yourself into a new way of thinking than it
is to think yourself into a new way of acting.

—Millard Fuller

Whenever I overhear my husband chatting on the phone, I can, with close to 100 percent accuracy, determine who is on the other end of the line. After twenty-plus years, I know him well enough to recognize tone and colorful lexicon, who receives formal language, and who warrants the more familiar, testosterone-infused, *yeah, man*. And though, as a therapist, I am trained to be tuned in to word choice, intonation, and inflection, this ability is not unique to me, nor is the switching up of changeable personas unique to my husband. This identity fluctuation does not mean he is disingenuous, suffering from what was once referred to as multiple personality disorder, or a big fat faker. Rather, his modification in personality, common to us all, can be explained by what psychologists refer to as *ego states*.

Ego states are a related pattern of feelings, thoughts, experience, and behaviors from either childhood or adulthood that, combined, affect our current interactions and perceptions. To simplify, ego states are the particular personality traits that emerge in specific situations and with certain people and together compose who we are as a whole. For example, how I am around my six-year-old differs from how I relate to a client in therapy or when out with my friends. Though I am completely authentic in each scenario, I may act more silly, playful, serious, or laid-back, depending on the situation and with whom I am interacting. We all, to some degree, alter our personalities automatically and unconsciously. Adapting to suit the needs and nuances of each relationship, as long as it originates from a genuine place, enables us to connect and communicate efficiently.

In some ego states we feel at ease and full of confidence, while in others we suffer from what is called the *imposter syndrome*, a psychological term for the experience of self-doubt in a particular situation. The imposter syndrome is triggered by uncertainty, new experiences, and doubts regarding our competence. In case you thought it was just you, that there exists a well-established psychological nomenclature proves its universality. The imposter syndrome includes that convincing voice in our head declaring that we are out of our league, that we have no idea what we are doing, or that if someone finds out how incompetent and clueless we really are, we will be fired on the spot. These exaggeratedly pessimistic thoughts naturally engender worry, fear, anxiety, and paralysis, which is precisely why it is crucial we notice their arrival. If we are inattentive to the potential power of the imposter syndrome, self-doubt and shame are perpetuated, inevitably stunting our abilities and growth.

When we are aware of which ego state embodies confidence and empowerment, however, we can use this to our advantage and apply these skills to areas in which we do not feel so self-assured. By mentally transferring positive attributes from one area of our lives to another, we borrow from the familiar personality strengths in one ego state to shore up our confidence in another when that mischievous little imposter syndrome shows up. For example, you might be fearless in your personal life when standing up for yourself with your partner but struggle with assertiveness at work. Likewise, I work with clients who feel self-assured and at the top of their game at the office but dissolve into a disorganized, insecure mess on the home front. My own comfort zone, or ego state, is in one-on-one interactions with others. I feel confident and at ease when working individually with clients. Though I am continually growing and am certainly imperfect, I am also compassionate, seasoned, and possess a wealth of information. My public-speaking ego state, on the other hand, is not so self-assured.

The Ego States Mindful Break allows us to transfer our skills from our comfort zone in order to lessen the uneasiness and insecurity in an undesirable ego state. In practice, I can borrow some of that treasured confidence from my therapist ego state when commanding center stage. As in a session, I focus on just one person at a time and speak directly to her. This not only serves to remind me of our shared experience dealing with stress and overwhelm but also brings me back into my comfort zone—that ego state of one-on-one. This is not a cure-all quick fix, though it is a welcome respite from that persistent, naysaying imposter and provides a shot of reassurance, to boot.

Similarly, when that old, unproductive imposter syndrome creeps into my writing space, I greet it dispassionately and, instead, usher the familiarity of the individual therapy relationship into the creative process. It often feels intimidating and overwhelming to think about reaching *all women* with my prose; rather, I can imagine writing to one singular woman, addressing her personally, thereby lessening the enormity of the endeavor. (When facing such creative self-doubt, see the U-Shaped Curve Mindful Break, page 227.)

Lest I paint an entirely unfavorable picture of our defenseless imposter—and before it starts to develop a complex, maybe even suffering from its own imposter syndrome (oh, the irony)—it must be noted that its appearance can serve us well by galvanizing us to take a genuine look at the underpinnings of our insecurities. Perhaps we improve our knowledge and abilities; maybe we identify a few concrete ways in which we can enhance our confidence with additional training or experience. To gain public speaking experience and self-confidence, for instance, I may join Toastmasters, read up on the topic, or hire a speaking coach.

When it comes to an objective assessment of true deficits, it may be beneficial to enlist a trusted friend to assist you, as research shows women tend to minimize and downplay their own wisdom and capabilities. The Ego States Mindful Break supports our performance and enhances our confidence until we fill in the proficiency gaps, if truly needed.

It is important to distinguish between culling true strengths from our confident ego states and pretending to be someone we are not. Transferring skills from one state to another is only effective if we are authentic in our interactions with others and honest with ourselves in fully owning our shortcomings. The more genuine we are, the less energy we expend on covering up our self-perceived flaws. Naming and owning the imposter not only frees up our precious energy for bigger and better things but also invites others to do the same. Creativity, innovation, and effort can then be freely spent on the work itself rather than exhaustedly wrestling with that old imposter in our head.

The Ego States Mindful Break

❶ Identify areas of your life or circumstances in which you feel most proud or self-assured. Here is where you will find your confident ego states.

❷ What are the specific strengths utilized in this ego state? Perhaps, as a friend, you are loyal, kind, and an especially good, nonjudgmental listener. At work you might be organized, reliable, and highly regarded as the go-to person for complicated projects.

❸ Notice areas where the imposter syndrome arises: When called to perform specific tasks at work? When in conversation with someone in your personal life? When the self-doubt is triggered, take care to note the negative chatter as simply the imposter doing its thing—not allowing the critical *thoughts* to morph into unsubstantiated *facts* in your mind (which occurs far more often than we realize).

❹ Imagine transferring those strengths from your confident ego states into those that are lacking. Remember, if all of those ego states are pieces of you, they exist within you all the time and are there for the taking.

❺ Finally, you may choose to share this mindful break with others in your organization. Being able to name fear and self-doubt reinforces that it is indeed a universal experience, destigmatizes its appearance, and allows for a more authentic, vulnerable workplace culture. Go slowly and be judicious with how much you share and with whom. Above all else, start with being honest, kind, and compassionate with yourself.

Don't Forget to Play

The opposite of play isn't work. It's depression.

—Jane McGonigal

Adulting is hard. And exhausting. As busy women we're often so intent on taking care of business that we allot scant time for pure amusement. Though some of us have managed to fiercely hang on to a sense of play, most struggle to merely recall what it is we once did for fun.

Even for adults, playing is vital to our well-being. But how do we do this when we have aged out of playgrounds and imaginary worlds? According to research, "Playfulness can be defined as an internal predisposition characterized by creativity, curiosity, pleasure, sense of humor, and spontaneity. This attitude extends to all life situations and modifies how adults perceive, evaluate, and approach situations." So, playfulness infuses all aspects of our lives. It also enables us to "approach situations with an open mind to find original solutions to problems, to confront difficulties, and to accept failure."[20] The upside is that even if we are not inherently inclined toward a playful nature, what we practice grows stronger—the more we play, the more playful we become.

Humor, levity, and fun are necessary life ingredients not only to compensate for all that grown-up seriousness but also to counteract work–life imbalance, stress, and

Without play, we might never be able to make the unexpected connections that are the essence of insight.
—Anne-Marie Slaughter

even boredom. Take Jen, for example, a work-from-home customer service rep whose job responsibilities are understimulating but pay the mortgage and provide invaluable flexibility—which are important for her as a single mom. To offset the workweek boredom, Jen schedules lively weekend outings with her young school-age daughter and friends. Hiking, kayaking, and pottery painting with her daughter fulfill her.

For me, frolicking outside is the ticket; when my inner child shows up, stress happily slips away. A while back I joined Colleen Cannon, former world champion triathlete and founder of Women's Quest, and an enthusiastic group of women for a fall adventure retreat full of hiking and biking. Although comfortable on two wheels, I had never mountain biked down winding, roots- and rock-covered single-track trails. Until Women's Quest.

I learned that it is strangely comforting and grounding when I focus on pushing myself out of my comfort zone (careering down a black diamond mountain bike trail) and someone in front (that would be Colleen) playfully exclaims, *"Wheeeeeee!"* My shoulders are allowed to relax and drop. A brilliantly delivered reminder to *have fun* while fearing for our lives is instrumental during the intense concentration of learning a new skill. Challenging myself in this way was simultaneously frightening and exhilarating. I came home feeling like a warrior, ready to tackle any hurdle along my path.

Stepping out of our comfort zones in new ways to play is empowering and translates into confidence in other areas of our lives. There are infinite ways to have fun and be adventurous, certainly not all requiring mortal danger and adrenaline. Creating time for what fills us up is crucial, however, to a balanced, joy-filled life. So go on out there and play!

The Don't Forget to Play Mindful Break

If you regularly partake in a handful of playful hobbies, you've got this mindful break covered. Good for you! Keep it up and be sure to expand your repertoire.

❶ Maybe you are fully aware of beloved playful activities but need to recommit to inking them into your schedule. If so, identify two and decide right now where, when, and with whom you will engage.

❷ Unleash your inner child. Though you may be out of practice, if you once embodied playfulness as a kid, the capacity is still there waiting to be reignited.

3 If you have no idea how you would even begin to play, choose a single activity and try it once. Experiment. Keep an open mind. You never have to do it again if it doesn't suit.

4 What have you always wanted to try? What activity have you wished you knew how to do? Some ideas to get you started: Go zip-lining. Paint and sip. Learn a musical instrument. Take a dance class. Go ice skating. Cultivate a garden. Try geocaching. Craft jewelry. Go bird watching.

5 If you are prone to seriousness or hang on tightly when learning a new skill, be sure to intentionally veer toward a more lighthearted and amusing tone.

6 Use well-intentioned humor at work when appropriate. Share funny anecdotes. Smile, laugh, connect. Purposefully infuse the workplace with measured playfulness.

7 Step back and view the world with a more spirited lens. Search for levity and fun. Be serious when necessary; be playful when possible.

Why Not Me?

Fear is a natural reaction to moving closer to the truth.
—Pema Chodron

When we allow our dreams to expand outside our comfort zone, it can feel downright uncomfortable and over-whelming, as all sorts of real or imagined self-induced barriers arise. We may need to wade through a barrage of obstacles on our way to attainment of our dreams—from well-meaning folks with divergent advice to those not-as-well-meaning attempting to dissuade us to those who believe we've lost our minds for even trying. Of course, the loudest, most obnoxious voice asserting the countless reasons why we should not even bother can be the one in our very own head. (See also Your Inner Bully Mindful Break, page 140, for more evidence of this doubting voice.)

When we learn to expect, recognize, and accept the appear-ance of those barriers, we position ourselves in a place of empow-erment to continue on in spite of them. Take Samantha, for example. Though she had never run more than a neighborhood block in her life, she dreamed of running a 5K race with her friends. The following are some impediments she finds herself up against (and how she successfully addresses them):

Physical. As Samantha starts training (a bit too zealously at first), she begins to suffer from uncomfortable shin splints.

The antidote: Rather than falling to her knees, silently thanking the running gods for an excuse to bail out, Samantha continues to build fitness with cross-training (biking and yoga) until she is able to lace up those running shoes and get out there pain free once again.

> *You block your dream when you allow your fear to grow bigger than your faith.*
>
> —Mary Manin Morrissey

Logistical. Working a forty-plus-hour week, raising kids, and helping run a household leaves little time for exercise.

The antidote: Each Friday, Samantha schedules in her training for the week, reminding herself that even short, consistent exercise sessions are much better than none at all. This consists of everything from a brisk twenty-minute lunchtime walk at work to waking fifteen minutes early to get in some yoga, to an impromptu flag football game in the park with her children.

Psychological. As a child, Samantha was told by more than one adult that she was not the athletic type. She naively, but understandably, bought into that subjective judgment, internalized it, and has doubted her capacity to be a runner ever since. Negative self-talk such as, "I can't . . ." or "I'm not [fill in the blank] enough," is common and persuasive.

The antidote: Samantha searches for evidence that she is indeed athletic, breaks goals down into manageable micro-action steps (running a half mile without stopping), offers herself tons of high fives, and proudly shares her continuous effort and progress with family and friends. She also remains vigilant for those limiting beliefs, shifting them into positive self-affirmations by both faking it until she becomes it and with consistent *I can, I will* statements. Eventually, Samantha starts to believe it *and* become it, successfully completing her first 5K race.

So, whether your dream consists of a lofty career goal, the adoption of a simple healthy habit, or a long-held personally fulfilling objective, be sure to use the Why Not Me? Mindful Break to head off those limiting beliefs at the pass.

Why Not Me? Mindful Break

❶ Imagine I am sitting down across from you, looking straight into your eyes, kindly but firmly inquiring: *Why not you?* In other words, *I believe in you.*

❷ Identify the barriers. What are your *perceived* physical, logistical, and psychological limitations? Are there any others standing in your way?

❸ Is this limiting belief a thought or a fact?

❹ Decide how you will address or work around each of them. It may be helpful to enlist a trusted friend to assist you.

⑤ Consider what your dream or goal might look like if it were easy. Hang on to that vision of possibility in moments of struggle.

⑥ What would you do if you knew you would succeed?

⑦ What's the worst that can happen if you try? What's the best-case scenario? What about something in between?

When we learn to expect resistance and obstacles on the way to reaching our goals, we can outsmart our own limiting beliefs, potential distractions, overwhelm, and fear of failure (or of success). The self-doubt and fear can chatter on all it wants. Ultimately it is *you* who gets to choose whether or not you believe it. So, let's try that again: *Why not you?*

The Afternoon Slump
(aka Bellows Breath)

Stand up straight and realize who you are, that you tower over your circumstances.

—Maya Angelou

Have you ever had that experience of sitting in a dull lecture, the speaker droning on as you fought back near-painful sleepiness? Or that yawning, desperate attempt to keep your head from bobbing so as not to land facedown on your desk as sleep finally overtakes you at work?

Sometimes, despite my best efforts, I revisit the land of tormented grogginess in midafternoon. Rather than immediately resort to another cup of caffeinated buzz, I enlist the help of this mindful break meant to increase alertness and energy, which is exactly what I need to counteract that troublesome afternoon slump.

The Afternoon Slump Mindful Break[21]

This break can be a tad noisy. You may want to find a private place to practice, lest others overhear you and fear you are having a full-blown panic attack or are in the process of going postal. If you do not have your own office, the bathroom, stairwell, or supply closet will do just fine.

1 Sit or stand tall with the spine straight. Pause for a moment to notice the body sensations of tiredness. Is there a burning or heaviness in your eyes? Does your head feel foggy? Is there achiness in the body? Where? Simply notice without judgment.

2 Keeping your mouth closed yet relaxed, inhale and exhale as quickly as you can through the nose, with equal amount of force and duration. You might notice the muscles of the back of the neck, the chest, and abdomen tighten as you do. The goal is to mimic a bellow with the rapid movement of the diaphragm, ideally with three inhales and exhales per second.

3 Begin with ten to fifteen seconds, building up the amount of time by five seconds each time you practice, eventually working up to one minute. Allow the breath to settle into a normal pace after each cycle. Take care to not overdo it, especially if this is a brand-new-to-you practice.

4 Notice body sensations once again. What has changed? Do you sense an increase in energy? If so, where?

5 This may require a bit of practice before results are clear. Be patient and stay curious. Congratulate yourself for trying something new, noncaffeinated, and healthy.

6 Now get back to work, hopefully with a little more pep in your step.

Self-R-E-S-P-E-C-T

Each time a woman stands up for herself, she stands up for all women. —**Maya Angelou**

Anne Lamott, one of my favorite authors, writes about hosting a gathering of beloved friends at her home, and later in the evening, nearly instantaneously reaching a point when she is done—as in, *OK, everyone, time to go! I adore you all but I am ready for quiet, bed, and sleep.* To this, I can completely relate. I love to spend time with friends and family over a glass or two of wine, but as an early riser and natural introvert, I, too, hit a nighttime limit when I have run out of steam. My brain ceases to compute, my conversational ability screeches to a halt, and I yearn longingly for my bed. The difference between the two of us (besides her being a contemporary literary icon) is that while I merely fantasize about it, she announces to her friends when it is time to go. *Out loud.* (I know!)

You see, Anne Lamott is of that awesome breed of no-holds-barred honest women for whom scooting partygoers out of her house mid-gathering is not unexpected. She knows what she needs and is not afraid to own it and assert herself. Even better, people still love and respect her, quite likely because of it. Being able to recognize, accept, and kindly ask for what we need, even if it is not always popular or socially acceptable, is a rare, admirable trait. Ultimately, it is showing ourselves respect by honoring who we are at the core and using our voice to communicate it with courage. I, for one, am still working on this level of transparency. You can be quite confident, though, that if you are ever at my home on a Saturday night, 9:30 PM is about my limit for entertaining.

The Self-R-E-S-P-E-C-T Mindful Break

Know thyself. As you move through your days, pause and take a moment to recognize your likes, dislikes, and preferences. Some of us are more in tune with this than others. What tends to provide an overall sense of ease and lightness when thought about? These are your likes. What provokes a tense, restricted heaviness? These are your dislikes.

Own it and respect it. Accept and, dare I say, embrace these unique pieces of you. Know that you are worthy of them. As long as we are respectful of others in the process, our quirks can be endearing and allow for more authentic connection with others.

Ask for what you need. Try on those assertiveness skills. Use your body to garner confidence. Stand tall, take up more space, power pose, make eye contact.

Use a strong voice, lowering it a notch. Speak clearly, slowly, and with confidence (even if, at first, you are faking it until you become it).

R-E-S-P-E-C-T. Find out what it means to *you* and turn some of that goodness back onto yourself.

High Fives

—

Create an environment where people feel valued and appreciated for who they are, not just what they do.
—Mike Robbins

I recently had tea with my very first meditation teacher, now a longtime friend and mentor. Without Ali, I may never have begun meditating regularly and would never have met her writer husband, Roger, who graciously took the time to advise and edit, line by line, my first ever book proposal. Without their benevolent support, the countless opportunities that arose from the publication of my first book, *Breathe, Mama, Breathe*, would never have occurred. When it came time to compile the acknowledgments section, it was a wonderfully heartwarming practice to reflect on, and thank, all who contributed to this personal and professional milestone. Of course, including Ali and Roger among those thanked was a no-brainer.

Though it may, at first, seem as if we have accomplished a feat solo, there are always others who have supported our success in some way, if even indirectly. Pausing to reflect, we begin to comprehend the infinite nature of the list. Most of us are not routinely required to craft book acknowledgments, though perhaps we should be, as those small acts of gratitude, what I refer to as high fives, matter so much more than we realize.

I would maintain that thanks are the highest form of thought; and that gratitude is happiness doubled by wonder.

—G. K. Chesterton

Take Sara, for example. She's now a school administrator who taught second grade early in her career. As she was unassumingly choosing oranges at the grocery store one day a smiling young adult approached and introduced herself as a former student. This recent college grad proudly announced that it was because of Sara's encouraging influence that she had chosen to become a teacher. Not only did Sara tear up sharing the story with me, but upon hearing it, I experienced the secondhand warmth of appreciation as well. One spoken high five—what a ripple effect, what a gift.

When was the last time someone extended a sincere expression of gratitude to you? Too often we are the recipients of a gentle critique sandwich (at best) or blatant criticism (at worst). Likewise, when did you last offer a deep expression of gratitude to someone who has touched your life, made it easier, or provided an opportunity you may not have otherwise received? Rarely do we receive high fives about how we have helped improve the lives of others.

I write this not to induce guilt and pessimism but to share the feel-good benefits of expressing appreciation and gratitude. When we intentionally share the credit for our successes, those relationships are strengthened: The recipient feels appreciated and we, as the high-fiver, experience increased happiness as well. Positive reinforcement is motivating. Research shows that in the workplace gratitude is linked "to more positive emotions, less stress and fewer health complaints, a greater sense that we can achieve our goals, fewer sick days, and higher satisfaction with our jobs and our coworkers."[22]

High fives are such simple, small investments of time and energy that cultivate potentially far-reaching benefits by highlighting those micro-successes. There are infinite opportunities to offer gratitude to those we work and live with. Let's champion and support one another, lifting each other up with those powerful high fives.

The High Fives Mindful Break

Perhaps stating the obvious, the appreciation must be sincere. If you are struggling with identifying any positive qualities or actions of your colleagues, carve out a bit of time for self-reflection. If we search carefully enough, we can find value in nearly everyone. (See also Kindness Mindful Break, page 55.)

❶ Think of someone you appreciate, how you were impacted by that person, and what gratitude toward them feels like. Then send the person a note, e-mail, or text expressing your thanks.

❷ Take the next five minutes to select three people, one at a time, and tell those people three things you value about them.

❸ Write your acknowledgments page—whether for assistance on a specific work project, some long-ago meaningful influence, or in regard to your career in general. List all the people who contributed to your success and outline specifically how they did so. Then let them know.

❹ Develop a High Five Mindful Break peer recognition program at your workplace. Some organizations have a bulletin board full of high-five Post-it Notes, others start meetings with colleague high fives. Include everyone in this happiness project.

❺ Notice what has changed in your mood, relationships, and worldview after practicing this mindful break.

What Are Your Superpowers?

Life can be much broader once you discover one simple fact, and that is that everything around you that you call "life" was made up by people no smarter than you.

—Steve Jobs

Superpowers. We all have them. Each of our own unique combination of strengths adds up to some serious influence and talent, though a number of barriers can prevent us from harnessing them to our full advantage. Perhaps we have never given them much consideration as we plug away at the daily grind. Maybe we were raised to believe we must remain humble above all else. Or, as is common, we spend most of our precious mental energy focused on the plethora of our perceived deficits rather than assets.

In a world that seems to laud and reward outgoing, outspoken extroverts, for example, I had always believed my quiet, introverted nature to be a disadvantage in need of remediation. I felt this especially in the business realm, despite that my natural inclination to listen and observe is precisely part of what makes me excel at my work—as therapist and coach; as a solitary, silent writer; and when happily turning the spotlight over to clients or colleagues through collaboration or mentoring. It has taken me many years, plenty of self-empowerment coaching work, and interactions with a few quietly powerful women to perceive these traits as my own unique superpowers.

We need to allow ourselves to recognize those positive traits and strut them out! In order to be your best self, employee, boss, wife, mother, friend, citizen, and any other role you can imagine, you need to rock those strengths. The world needs you—the rest of us women need you—to utilize and harness what only you can bring. So let's get to it.

What Are Your Superpowers? Mindful Break

From the list below, select your strengths, either circling them or writing them down in a notebook. You need not embody these qualities all the time—no one does. Choose based on which you exhibit when at your best. Now is not the time for humility. Pick as many as you'd like and feel free to add your own to the list:[29]

Fair. Leaderly. Cautious. Humble. Prudent. Optimistic. Creative. Integrity. Loving. Critical thinker. Courageous. Loyal. Team player. Honest. Zestful. Generous. Disciplined. Faithful. Hopeful. Curious. Brave. Persistent. Loving. Wise. Kind. Gritty. Energetic. Funny. Spiritual. Playful. Grateful. Forgiving. Strong. Resilient. Intelligent. Athletic.

If you find this challenging (or even if you don't), ask a few trusted friends or family members which traits they would choose for you when you are at your personal best and why.

Reflect on situations, both at work and out in the world, when you have exhibited these superpowers. Notice accompanying body sensations, if any.

Create your list and keep it visible. Combine a few to create a new password to be reminded of them frequently. Place them on your computer screen saver. Place a sticky note on your desk at work or your bathroom mirror at home. Own those strengths. Consider how they contribute to your success.

Revisit your list periodically to update it, if necessary, and keep adding to your inimitable arsenal of superpower work and life applications.

Feel the Burn

I had to decide to stay upright on my surfboard. I didn't know it would help me stay upright in my life, too.
—Eve Fairbanks

This mindful break is especially for those who have not, historically, been huge fans of exercise. Wait! Before you turn the page, I'd like to invite you to consider exercise in a brand-new way—simply as moving your body with enjoyment. If until this point you have been an avowed non-exerciser I imagine you might be rolling your eyes. I dare you to try it for just a few days. For those of you who are already avid fans, Feel the Burn is an invitation to get curious, increase self-awareness, and up your mental game.

I have a friend who has run several one-hundred-mile trail races (not a typo!) up and down mountains—without sleeping and only stopping to quickly eat, drink, and relieve himself—*for fun*. No one is chasing him, there is no massive monetary or fame-inducing prize and no tangible reward save his own sense of satisfaction, pride, and bragging rights. *Why?* I have asked him, sincerely attempting to understand his otherworldly motivation and perseverance. Although I love all sorts of physical activity, including trail running, I have zero desire to push myself to anywhere near those limits. I prefer to watch, fascinated from afar as I observe and unpack what drives such extremes.

When it comes to ultra-athletes' endurance, there must be some level of distraction and grit and also a clear answer as to why. *Why in the world should I keep going?* The best answer I've received from my friend is that he loves to see what he is capable of—that's enough for him. My motivation for exercise has more to do with my love of being outside, getting my heart pumping, and the delicious aftereffects. (See also Afterburn Mindful Break, page 195.)

Regardless of where you fall on the exercise continuum, there are lessons to be learned from such physical high achievers. By embracing their deftly honed mindful performance tools we can transform our perception of mild physical unpleasantness— learning to accept and even welcome it—and allow ourselves the ability to progress and persist.

To understand this mindfulness tool consider what qualifies some sensations as acceptable, even satisfying, and others as painful. Plain and simple: perception. With mindfulness, we step back to consider that, pleasant or unpleasant, they are all simply sensations. For example, sometimes when I'm out running, chronic sciatic nerve pain rears its ugly head, sending electric zaps down my leg, straight into my foot. When I experience these uncomfortable sensations, my body's (and mind's) natural reaction is to tense and resist. When I bring awareness to the sensations themselves, I breathe deeply, relax those tight muscles, and, with curiosity and acceptance (rather than judgment), observe the nuances. *Dull ache, tingling, periodic zapping and stabbing, slight burning.* As I continue to notice, I also realize the subtle sensations shift in intensity and duration. It is not a fixed situation, therefore neither is my perception. When categorized as pain, I tense and resist. When thought of as merely sensations, I more readily accept.

I can, if I so choose, deliberately turn my attention away from the sciatica and onto something more appealing, say the birds singing or the smell of fallen leaves. This is in direct contrast to attempting to ignore the discomfort. Instead, I recognize it and *choose* whether to maintain focus on it.

If you're a newbie exerciser, you may feel a bit of discomfort at the outset. This is normal, but please keep it to a minimum. There is an important distinction between discomfort that should be heeded (injury or overdoing it) and unpleasantness due to unfamiliar movements, pace, or activity. The point is to get you moving in a way that feels wonderful for your body, in whatever way makes sense for you—strolling in the park, Zumba, ice skating, gentle yoga—not pushing so hard you are unable to climb out of bed the next day. Experiment with nudging yourself out of your comfort zone firmly and kindly. Ultimately, Feel the Burn should burn in only the best of ways.

Feel the Burn Mindful Break

It's important to check in with your doctor before beginning any new exercise program. Do that.

1 First, think of three reasons *why* you are going to move your body with enjoyment. Even better, write them down on index cards and place them where they are visible. For example, increased energy, feeling better in your clothes, staying healthy for your family, stress relief, or the long-held unfulfilled desire to consider yourself an athlete.

2 Know where you fall on the physical self-challenging spectrum so you can nudge or back off accordingly. If it has been some time since you've gotten the old ticker pumping, take it slowly. (See 5-Minute Walk, page 95.)

3 Plan it out. Each Sunday, map out the week ahead. Write down the day and time, and what type of exercise you will engage in. As you become more skilled, check in with yourself each day to assess what type of movement your body is craving. (If you develop a feel-the-burn habit, you will indeed crave it!)

4 Observe the sensations and attendant thoughts nonjudgmentally. If your inner chatter starts to resemble a mean old drill sergeant, switch that voice to one that would encourage your best friend. If you experience slight physical discomfort, play around with noticing it, breathing deeply, relaxing into it, and persisting.

5 Afterward, tune in to any shifts in sensation, changes in posture, and where you feel more alive. Remember those positive changes and come back to them when you are questioning your *why*.

Ultimately, respect your body. Challenge yourself with kindness rather than employing a punitive stance. Move so that it feels good and you keep coming back for more—and don't be surprised when one day you discover you have created an enduring love for feeling the burn.

Afterburn

I've learned that how I look and feel is important to me, for reasons beyond health and vanity. It may sound clichéd, but it's true: If I'm confident, people are more likely to listen to me. If more people are listening, I have more power to fight effectively for what I believe in.

—Senator Kirsten Gillibrand

It's 5:15 AM on a frigid, dark winter morning. Snuggled and toasty warm in my bed, I tentatively reach out from under the five layers of covers to shut off the increasingly loud beep of my ancient alarm clock. Today, predawn is the only available time in the schedule for exercise. The cold tip of my nose forewarns of the chilly temperature in the house, tempting me to burrow more deeply into the coziness, switch off the alarm, and drift happily back into dreamland.

No, wait! I also know how amazing it will feel once I'm up, dressed, and stretched out on my yoga mat, body and breath synching gratefully. I will be more clearheaded, awake, creative, and happy. I will walk taller, shoulders pulled back, with a natural boost of confidence. I will be a kinder mom, wife, and therapist.

Precisely because of such countless benefits accrued over the years, I find the wherewithal to throw off the soft comforters, venture into the frosty bathroom, and, finally, onto my well-worn yoga mat.

I make no apologies for the fact that I am downright selfish when it comes to making time to exercise. Each Sunday, after sketching out the week's work schedules, kids' activities, and other commitments, exercise is next to be penciled in. Actually, I ink it in, and I guard it carefully. It's my self-protection from burnout, from both mental and physical lethargy, and from the busyness that can easily creep in and take over if I allow it. Having said that, I have also learned to be flexible in how and when I carve out the time.

Some days, if there is enough morning light to run outdoors, I lace up my shoes, throw back a few swigs of coffee, munch two bites of banana, and head out for a run before I barely even register what is happening. Once home, I stretch, shower, grab the rest of the coffee and, at times, question if I actually ran that three-mile loop in my half-awake stupor.

I do occasionally run in the morning darkness, but only when I need to be at the top of my game. If you catch me out running on the predawn country roads with my canine companion, the glow of the awkward headlamp bouncing with every step, chances are that I have a speaking engagement later that morning. Forty-five minutes of flow yoga works, too, but for me, there is nothing like the fresh air and heart-pumping of feet on the pavement. As I focus on the road, breath, and body, inspired ideas arise organically and pick up speed, from a mere trickle to a creativity fountain. Afterward, I feel alive, grateful, and pumped up with endorphins. And that, my friend, is the afterburn of which I speak. I am not only fully awake, but also more mentally alert and imaginative.

What I experience is now supported by research that shows exercise appears to enhance creativity, independent of mood.[23] According to the American Psychological Association, exercise also reduces symptoms of anxiety, depression, and stress by encouraging your bodily systems—such as the one that controls heart rate and respiration and the one responsible for movement—to communicate in making sure you are coping competently with emotional and physical challenges. "This workout of the body's communication system may be the true value of exercise; the more sedentary we get, the less efficient our bodies in responding to stress."[24] According to Gretchen Reynolds, in *The New York Times* Well blog, vigorous exercise has also been shown to increase the protein called brain-derived neurotrophic factor (BDNF), which appears to play a particular role in improving memory, recall, and skilled task.[25]

Regardless of how many speeches and workshops I offer, I still start out nervous. It's no wonder I have intuitively used exercise to calm my nerves, up my creativity, and sharpen my performance. If the research isn't convincing enough, I urge you to test out the Afterburn Mindful Break for yourself.

The Afterburn Mindful Break

This break is about tuning in to your body, posture, mood, and level of confidence after exercise. Ideally, you will engage in aerobic heart-pumping activity. However, if you are a non-exerciser, start small and build up over time. Five minutes of brisk walking can definitely do the trick.

1 Choose a form of movement and get your heart pumping for a minimum of five minutes.

2 What do you notice post-movement? Are you more patient and tolerant as you commute to work? More quick-witted and mentally sharp? Funnier? More playful? Is your energy increased and sustained throughout the day? Are you happier and more content? Do you naturally stand taller? If positive outcomes are not immediately noticeable, don't fret. I guarantee they will show up over time, sometimes subtly. Keep going.

3 Jot down your observations in a notebook, as this can be useful to compare progress and motivate ourselves for more.

4 Build on the length and intensity of exercise and continue to enjoy the perks of moving your body with appreciation and delight.

Who Am I Becoming?

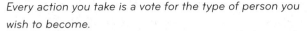

Every action you take is a vote for the type of person you wish to become.

—James Clear

Considering the mixed messages we receive about how to prevail as a successful modern woman, it's no wonder thoughts about our own appearance can be paradoxical at times—do we stroll into the networking event donning comfortable, practical flats or suffer in those power pumps all night?

We all create narratives about ourselves, including our appearance—some unconscious and long-standing, some rooted in a clear external source, some self-inflicted, and most absolutely unfounded. Consider something as simple as makeup. Women run the gamut from never-leave-home without a fully made-up face to never having wielded a mascara wand in their lives. Years ago I unintentionally cultivated a belief that in order to be perceived as professionally competent I must adorn my face with cosmetics. My personal makeup narrative was solidified in the fact that as a twentysomething recent grad I appeared significantly younger than my age, which, although lovely in some ways, was not conducive to being taken seriously. *What can this inexperienced twenty-year-old possibly offer as a therapist?* I imagined some clients wondered upon meeting me for the first time. A dash of eyeliner and mascara added a few years to my youthful face, rendering me instantly more credible. Not an unreasonable rationale, in my estimation.

When I examine my history a bit further, however, I realize the fixed cosmetic routine began in earnest much earlier, as an easily influenced preteen emulating the world of teen magazines. My daily routine was only further strengthened when I underwent surgery to treat benign skin growth and was left with a prominent scar encircling my left cheek. It wasn't so much that I was ashamed of the disfigurement (though I'd prefer it wasn't there) but more that I was actually worried about the discomfort I imagined those forced to witness the angry-looking scar experienced, especially during those first few months post-op. So, the makeup habit endured, and each morning I devoted ten minutes to cosmetic application before heading out to the office.

Within the past year, however, I began leaving for work sans makeup. The change came about gradually, not so much out of an enlightened, feminist statement, but of merely growing tired of spending those precious few minutes applying makeup in the morning only to remove it some twelve hours later. I no longer wanted to be bothered. In its own small way, it also felt liberating, like owning who I am, embellishment-free—for a few pleasant seconds, that is; until the mind chatter commenced: *Are my clients wondering what's up with the disturbingly pallid complexion and dark under-eye circles? Are they imagining a serious illness, worried for my overall health, speculating as to why I look so god-awful? Is this distracting from their focus on treatment? Clearly it is distracting me.* Then, ushering myself back to rational thought, I recognized that, realistically, they never give it one iota of consideration. (Oh, that's right. The world does not revolve around me—except it does revolve around each of us in all of our minds, at times.)

Life isn't about finding yourself. Life is about creating yourself.
—George Bernard Shaw

And so, with my cautiously naked face, I alternate between feeling free—wholly myself, without need to disguise the flaws—and feeling sympathy for those forced to gaze at the under-eye greenish cast situated below two sadly sparse sets of eyelashes. Ultimately, I settle on the fact that, either way, people will acclimate. Slowly, my narrative has shifted. (Did you notice there is now zero concern about appearing too young to be taken seriously? That ship has definitely sailed. *Sniff-sniff.*)

I am not interested in dictating which specific life options you choose, least of all regarding makeup. If you relish spending thirty minutes beautifying your face because *you love it* (and not to meet anyone else's expectations) then, girl, you do you. I want nothing more than for you to feel gorgeous. When you feel beautiful, you also feel empowered and, most likely, *act* more powerful and confident.

I am also aware that my mascara tale may seem frivolous and inconsequential. Most of us have bigger fish to fry, I know. I share it, though, because it is a simple example of how our narratives about who we are and have been up to this point can remain fixed and unquestioned, with zero thought to the possibility that we are free to change at any time. Makeup is just *one* of the infinite pressures we women face and speaks to the precious energy, time, and thought expended on matters of societal expectation.

Who Am I Becoming? Mindful Break

The Who Am I Becoming? Mindful Break builds awareness of our true desires. Are my toenails painted that deep shade of red because it pleases me or because of societal expectations? It's a fine line between what we are choosing for ourselves and when we are caving to others' notions of how to be a woman. It is vital that we examine the underlying motivation and uncover the outdated narratives we hold about ourselves and who we *should be* so that we can decide consciously if they still resonate (if they were even truly our own ideas in the first place). There is no one right answer that fits all. In fact, yours may change and shift by the day. And that's OK. That's actually more than OK, as long as you are tuned in to what the reality is for you, which is where mindful awareness serves us well and real wisdom lies.

❶ What are some fixed ideas about who you are? (The smart one, the good listener, the reliable one, shy, loud, nerdy, disorganized, unathletic, fashionable?) Consider where and from whom those narratives developed.

❷ Do they still serve you well? If not, which would you like to change? What is the narrative you would prefer? How, specifically would that look?

❸ What is holding you back?

❹ Offer permission to reinvent yourself whenever you'd like. There is no right way, as long as you are staying true to yourself.

❺ You can create an identity, become a new, yet authentic version of yourself at any time. Be bold, be courageous. *Who are you becoming?*

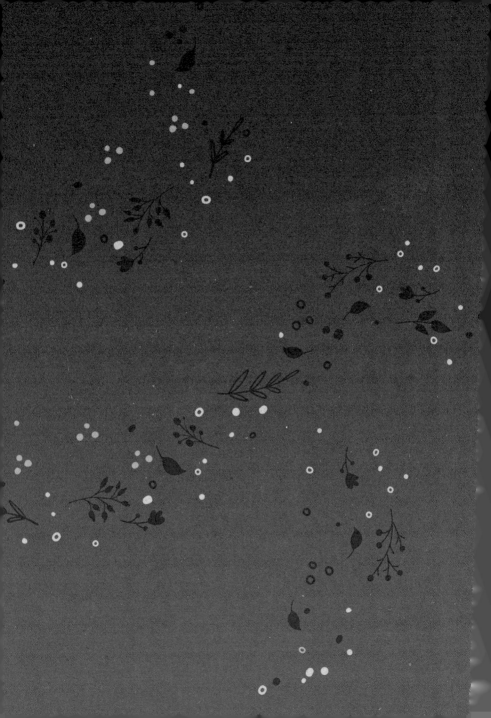

CHAPTER 3

Balance Mindful Breaks

Now that you have de-stressed and deepened your mindful awareness with the Breathe Mindful Breaks and boosted your awesomeness with the Becoming Mindful Breaks, it is time to create ongoing, sustainable balance in your life. As we do, it is vital that we remain intentional about what we take on and the direction we are headed. Without forethought and deliberate action, we can end up unwittingly spinning our wheels in a futile effort to put out the never-ending fires thrown our way. We can overdo and overcommit, inadvertently striving for *someone else's* idea of success rather than our own, and burn ourselves out in the process.

The Balance Mindful Breaks are intentional actions and periods of rest. They teach us how to identify and stay true to our deepest values as we move toward—and maintain—relative equilibrium. They allow us to dream big while breaking down those lofty aspirations into manageable micro-action steps, and encourage us to enjoy the journey along the way. The Balance Mindful Breaks help us recognize what can be delegated or let go, and what we can carve out more time for in our full lives. They are about prioritizing and taking care of ourselves while crafting a full, engaged life. With small, simple shifts, the Balance Mindful Breaks are ultimately about creating the absolute best version of ourselves and unleashing our unique combination of superpowers on the world.

Your Inner Compass (Identifying Core Values)

Be a good ancestor.   **—Marian Wright Edelman**

When we are so busy that our days run on automatic pilot, there is little time for connection, compassion, deep consideration of others, or consciously living by our values. The frantic pace leaves scant bandwidth for anything outside ourselves and our swirling thoughts. Inevitably, there are periods in our lives when, whether due to the burdensome or the wonderful, our cup runneth over, sending us into this definitively self-focused place. After writing and publishing *Breathe, Mama, Breathe*, for example, I was feeling a bit tunnel-visioned, with more of an all-encompassing focus on the project than I'd have liked. Although hugely grateful for the opportunity, the book writing, editing, planning, and promoting process consumed much of my time and capacity of mind. As my focus narrowed, so did my careful attention to some of my most deeply held values. Admittedly, I was not sprinting through my days committing random acts of *un*kindness, though this narrowed focus didn't sit well with me. While in the thick of it, I perceived a general sense of value unease, a nagging feeling that the balance was off, but the book and its attendant responsibilities would call to me, pulling me back in. It was not until the book launch hullabaloo had settled that I fully appreciated the extent of my drifting.

The conduct of our lives is the true reflection of our thoughts.
—Michel de Montaigne

We can remedy this sort of disconnection by deliberately reacquainting ourselves with our core values—what is most important to each of us. Fortunately, there are many ways to do this. One is the recent online trend of carefully selecting a single intentional word to usher in each New Year. Narrowing our choices down to just one word (any time of year) can help guide us as we face countless smaller choices. It's a sort of litmus test of what matters most when faced with various options: Do I say yes to this work project? How shall I spend a free afternoon? How might I best approach this challenging situation with my colleague? Does this choice move me in the direction of my deepest held values and my chosen word of intention?

Once *Breathe, Mama, Breathe* was written and out on bookshelves, I felt the pull to look up from my laptop, take in the wider world, and see where I could be of use: what I could do for others, how I could share what I have learned through the process. I chose that year's word to help guide me once again and landed on the value of . . . love.

At the time, in early 2017, love seemed to be fleeting in our society at large, if not completely absent. I wanted to meet fear with love. I wanted to meet anger with love, indifference with love, love with more love. If I approached each moment with love, I figured, everything else was covered. When we conjure up love, we are automatically more mindful, open, kind, compassionate, and grateful.

I knew this would be an imperfect endeavor, to say the least. I imagined a scenario in the not-too-distant future in which I'd lose my temper with my kids and experience that awful wash of shame and regret. I also knew that would be precisely when I would do my best to offer myself love and forgiveness, just as I strove to do with everyone else. I deliberately chose love for the whole year, allowing it to guide my decisions and interactions. As of this writing, *love* continues to top my list of values. Others on my list are *slow*, *nature*, and *growth*.

Identifying a short list of our most important values expands on this approach, giving us a clue as to where we would like to go. The alternative is to continually put out fires, constantly check off and add items to the to-do list, and run on that old, tiring automatic pilot. We need to be clear about our deepest-held values so they can guide us back on course when we have veered off unaware; our values are our life's compass.

Your Inner Compass Mindful Break

❶ Close your eyes, relax the body, and take three deep inhales and exhales, letting go of any expectations and shoulds. This is about staying true to yourself, not concerned with what you imagine others expect of you.

❷ If you need help, consult the list below and notice which words jump out at you. Which cause a subtle visceral reaction, maybe a lightness in the chest or a bit of increased energy overall? Have fun with it and feel free to create your own if something is missing from this list.

❸ Choose your top four values and write them down. Honesty. Health. Knowledge. Integrity. Family. Balance. Love. Play. Autonomy. Courage. Inspiration. Self-control. Authenticity. Giving back. Empathy. Faith. Soulfulness. Hope. Adventure. Forgiveness. Tradition. Growth. Success. Grit. Kindness. Generosity. Slowness. Freedom. Safety. Curiosity. Contentment. Pleasure. Wealth. Peace. Warmth. Prudence. Creativity. Simplicity. Security. Tolerance. Humor. Collaboration. Gratitude. Loyalty. Nature. Authority. Self-care. Achievement. Competition. Optimism. Happiness. Respect. Enthusiasm. Justice. Friendship. Compassion. Wisdom. Excellence. Humility. Flow.

❹ Why are those top four values important to you? Can you recall a time each played an important role in your life?

❺ Reflect on whether or how you are currently integrating your top core values into your home life. How about your work life? Which come easily to you and which might you spend more time focusing on? What gets in the way of living from your core values? What in your life could be altered in order to make this more of a reality? If self-judging arises (we recognize this when it contains shoulds or is accompanied by guilt), name it, gently sweep it aside, and remind yourself that you are working toward self-enhancement, offering yourself a high five instead.

❻ When facing a situation in which you are unsure or perplexed, refer back to your top values, using them as a guide to inform your decision.

When it comes to our values, it is important to perceive them as a helpful framework to create more of the life we want. The point is not to feel hemmed in by the values and resultant habits but instead to feel supported by them. If the framework begins to feel restrictive or pressured, step back and reassess your chosen values. Do they still resonate? What is the resistance about? Change is often uncomfortable. Don't mistake healthy growing pains as a sign that you are on the wrong track. Perhaps the structure needs some tweaking. Perhaps your top four values do, too. As we grow and change, so, too, might our top values, as they are a reflection of our priorities at any given time. Go back to review your list every so often, letting your wise, inner compass guide you.

Challenging People

—

Use the Teflon side of your mind, not just the Velcro side.
—Lama Surya Das

You know that one person in your life who, as you glimpse her walking toward you, elicits a subtle feeling of impending doom, an involuntary tightening of muscles, a silent scream of *Oh no, here she comes!?* Or whose incoming text or phone call causes your jaw to clench and stomach to execute a little flip-flop? If no one in your life fits this bill, you either live a blissfully hermit-like existence or can count yourself lucky. (If you have more than one, my sincere condolences—please spend some time with the Self-R-E-S-P-E-C-T, page 180, and High Fives, page 183, Mindful Breaks to buoy your own self-care, my friend.) For the rest of us, you know who I'm talking about—that challenging person who seems to suck the life out of us whenever we are in her presence for longer than thirty seconds, the mere thought of whom incites some low-level dread or a powerful desire to flee.

Perhaps this person is an occasional acquaintance or colleague with whom you must interact minimally, in which case you can steel yourself when with her, knowing the interaction will be short lived.

More formidable, however, is the unavoidable narcissistic sister-in-law, overly demanding superior, or consistently depressive next-door-neighbor. For better or worse, unless we divorce our partners, siblings, or our job itself (which may be the best option, in some cases), these folks are in our lives for good, so we might as well learn to coexist with them as graciously as possible.

I could fill an entire book on the whats, whys, and hows of challenging people and their various accompanying labels, diagnoses, and personality disorders. Sometimes our being faced with an energy vampire is immediately clear. Other times it is much subtler, requiring us to endure a few wearisome encounters before we recognize patterns and finally land on an *aha* moment, with full comprehension (and a touch of relief) that *it is not just me!* who feels this way around her. Suffice it to say, if after you engage in conversation with someone she walks away and you are left wondering *what in the world just happened* as you attempt to process the bewildering encounter, you are dealing with a difficult person. Other clues are marked deflation of your typically healthy sense of self-esteem or rapid triggering of your body's trusty fight-or-flight reaction.

It isn't only the seriously challenging people who drain our energy; you may have the sweetest, most hyperactive pal whose friendship you highly value but who also exhausts you if you spend too much time together. Likewise, those who put us slightly on edge exact a higher expenditure of energy—be it a micromanaging superior, a competitive colleague, or an occasionally tumultuous personal relationship. Each of these interactions require us to increase our awareness, tread lightly, and offer a large dose of kindness to ourselves.

If you are reading this and start to consider, *Could she be talking about* me? *Do others feel that way about* me? The mere arising of this question allows me to confidently assert that *you* are not one of the difficult ones, for it is precisely those troublesome folks who do not seem to possess the tiniest inkling that this description could possibly be applied to them. So, no worries.

> *When we manage a flash of mercy for someone we don't like, especially a truly awful person, including ourselves, we experience a great spiritual moment, a new point of view that can make us gasp.*
>
> —Anne Lamott

I tend to give people the benefit of the doubt, search for the positive in each of us, appreciate our quirks, and expect that the vast majority are innately good and well meaning. As a result (and probably with some luck thrown in), I require only one hand to count the folks I have met who decidedly fit into this mindful break category. Each time I do, however, I am left temporarily stunned at the unpleasant reaction it precipitates within me.

In these cases, it is important to be vigilant about the potential danger of sliding into a condescending position. Take care not to regard the challenging person as a definitive "other" as if *we* (clearly more evolved and self-aware, ahem) *would never* act in such a self-centered fashion, which, of course, we all do occasionally. The Challenging People Mindful Break is not so much about the flaws of the other as it is about how best to maintain our own dignity, sense of calm, and self-respect when encountering those unavoidable, vexing personalities. I use this mindful break myself when necessary—to cope, to preserve precious sanity, and as an opportunity to practice compassion. I hope it helps you, as well.

The Challenging People Mindful Break

1 Recognize when you are facing a challenging person. Unconscious reactions include tightening muscles, thoughts of irritation or self-doubt, and perhaps even a bit of shock—especially on our first go-round. If you are already familiar with the demanding nature of this individual, there may be an intense, immediate stiffening as you automatically prepare for battle. Queasiness, stomach discomfort, and quickening of the breath are also quite common.

2 *Breathe, my friend, breathe.* Your breath is your friend. Inhale, exhale. When at all possible, do not, I repeat, *do not* speak, return that e-mail, or send that text until you have grounded yourself with the breath. Then tenderly relax those clenched muscles . . . and onward you go.

3 Accept that this person is in your life, perhaps to stay, minimally in this moment. The goal is to lessen the discomfort, not to disregard, ignore, or resist it.

4 Compassion, compassion, compassion. Offer a good dose to yourself first. Only after you have directed some kindness your way, can you touch on the other person's humanity. In reality, we never really know all that is going on for someone behind the scenes that may be contributing to her behavior. Might you silently offer her some compassion for her (real or imagined) struggle? Note that this does not at all equate with allowing her to treat you unkindly or take her off the hook for an injustice. (For further support in this area, head over to the Kindness Mindful Break, page 55.)

5 Now slip into your imaginary suit of Teflon armor in order to take care of and protect yourself in the process. This suit is surprisingly light and effective, allowing plenty of room to breathe within. With challenging folks, it is especially necessary to maintain healthy emotional and physical boundaries. I like to imagine that when the negativity is flung my way, it slides effortlessly down that Teflon shield while I remain blissfully untouched on the other side. Your protective armor also prevents you from taking responsibility for someone else's emotional baggage, particularly when they've attempted to place it solely upon you.

6 Are there any lessons that can be gleaned from your interaction? Though it may seem virtually impossible in the moment, anytime we can pause and step back to observe, we have unhooked ourselves from the insanity and gained wise perspective. If we are willing to search, there is always a valuable lesson to be found within. If nothing else, you have bravely survived to see another day. Congratulations and a high five to you.

Make It Happen

> *It had long since come to my attention that people of accomplishment rarely sat back and let things happen to them. They went out and happened to things.*
>
> **—Leonardo da Vinci**

On her way into work as the sun was rising, Amy, swallowing hard against the lump in her throat, was desperately fighting back tears. She took a few deep breaths in an attempt to pull herself together as she anticipated the early morning meeting she was set to lead. Her thoughts drifted to the scene that had played out at home just a few minutes prior.

Amy's typical morning routine—snoozing the alarm three times before leaping out of bed, rushing frantically around while barking orders at her children, and searching for missing, but necessary, items—was inefficient at best. On this particular morning it finally all came to a head. As she ran out the door, she and her husband had a pointless fight while the kids stormed off to the bus stop overwhelmed, unmoored, and without any semblance of a proper goodbye.

Driving down the highway, Amy felt a nauseating combination of guilt, anger, frustration, and exhaustion—all before 7:45 AM. That was the moment Amy decided she was finished with stressful, frantic mornings and was ready for a change. In the past, she had periodically fantasized about a calm, slower start to the workday. She had even identified her top values as love, family, and balance, but she was at a loss as to how to transform the morning chaos.

We won't make ourselves more creative and productive by copying other people's habits, even the habits of geniuses; we must know our own nature, and what habits serve us best.

—Gretchen Rubin

Amy identified two specific goals: Pack a healthy lunch the night before and wake ten minutes earlier each morning to meditate. Some days, an epic battle was waged against that snooze button. Quickly reminding herself of the loving, relaxed morning she so craved provided the push she needed.

Amy began to appreciate how much calmer her mornings felt when she started with a few minutes of quiet to listen to the birds sing, observe the sunrise, and inhale the intoxicating aroma of strong coffee brewing. After a week of early rising, Amy began to greet her family with a contented smile instead of an overtired growl. She was more composed, grateful, and energized. Amy discovered firsthand how one small positive change, over time, can increase exponentially of its own accord;

how one seemingly impossible tweak transforms into healthy routines. Savoring the peace at home and enjoying a homemade healthy lunch at work, she soon found herself willingly replacing the sugar-crash-inducing donut typically scarfed down for breakfast at the office with a bowl of warm blueberry oatmeal enjoyed mindfully in her kitchen, where she perched happily by the open window.

As we identify goals, it is important to keep in mind that their purpose is to guide us, not to be rigidly followed at all costs and without periodic intentional revisions. Life sometimes takes us in a different direction, which is fine as long as we continue to filter those goals through our most deeply held values. (See also Your Inner Compass, page 207 to identify values). The Make It Happen Mindful Break outlines the steps to help you reach those goals one small positive change at a time.[26]

The Make It Happen Mindful Break

1 What do you want to accomplish? Be as specific as possible. Are your goals in alignment with your values? Make sure it is *your* goal, not a "should" generated by another influence.

2 What are your reasons for choosing this accomplishment? *Why* make this change? Imagine you have six months to live. What and who become most important? How do you spend your time? What falls away? What remains are your values and your *why*, helping to sustain motivation when the going gets tough.

❸ What are the micro-action steps needed? Begin with a verb, an action word. Break down the goal into the smallest possible micro-changes and bookend them between two already established habits. Create a goal that is attainable, but also demands some effort in order to keep it challenging.

❹ When will you work on them? When will they be completed? How will you fit these micro-changes into your schedule? Be specific and clear about what time, which days, and how often this will happen. Leave no room for ambiguity. Name target start and end dates.

❺ Who will help you get there? Whose assistance might be required?

❻ What roadblocks might get in your way? How will you deal with them? Expect resistance, address it, and recommit to your goal. When you face a setback or reach a plateau, notice the limiting negative thoughts. How would you support someone you cared about in getting back on track? Be firm yet kind with yourself.

❼ How will you know your plan is working? What are some specific measures of progress? It is easy to lose sight of the progress we've made when we are in the middle of change. Offer yourself plenty of positive encouragement for the beneficial micro-changes you make along the way.

8 With whom can you share your plan to keep you accountable? Who will cheer you on and not allow you to give up when the going gets tough?

9 Despite our persistence and best efforts, your goals may play out differently than planned. Keep moving toward them, remaining grounded in your values, in whatever wise direction seems plausible, regardless of the obstacles that arise. Where there's a will, there's a way.

10 Savor your hard-earned success, staying mindful of the process along the way.

The Green-Eyed Monster

*Do not spoil what you have by desiring what you have not;
remember that what you now have was once among the
things you only hoped for.*

—Epicurus

There are those workday mornings when the kids are en route to their respective schools and I am dashing out the door to my car, loaded down like a modern-day Sherpa with briefcase, handbag, and lunch box dangling precariously from my shoulders. As I pull out of the driveway, I glance over at my good friend and neighbor as she strolls back home from the bus stop, coffee mug in hand and ambling dog in tow. We each wave and extend a genuine smile goodbye. As I catch my breath and settle in for the short commute, I notice an uncomfortable tug of envy in my chest, as jealous thoughts begin to bubble up inside. *Man, I would love to have time in my schedule to meander about with the household chores, lie down for an afternoon nap should the urge arise, peruse a magazine while sipping tea, and relish the freedom from deadlines, work schedules, and infinite e-mails.*

I detect the emergence of envy for my friend's relaxed pace, the fresh air and sunshine I imagine she has all morning to bask in, the stay-at-home-mom-of-school-age-children schedule wide open in front of her until her kids arrive home some seven and half hours later. Sheepishly, I catch myself, sigh, and coax my mind back to reality and the literal road in front of me, and then I commence the self-judgment. *What is wrong with you?* I admonish. *You know her life is not all free time and bonbons nibbled decadently on the couch.* I do know. This current object of envy is also one of my very best friends. She is an attentive, loving, carpooling mom (to three active kids) who also single-handedly keeps her household operating smoothly.

Hold on there, Shonda! my inner voice of reality booms firmly but kindly, *you know exactly what this is about.* For better or worse, the green-eyed monster of envy is not unfamiliar to me, creeping in every so often when my life balance has tilted too far in one direction. Thankfully, though, I have learned to recognize its appearance as an invaluable source of information if I am willing to examine it, and myself, with honesty. Though unpleasant and powerful, envy can also clue us in to what is missing in our lives. Lo and behold, here is that green-eyed monster again.

I ask myself, *What is it you are really craving?* The answer appears with surprising ease: *I crave free, open, unscheduled time.* Period. Not the imagined naps, not the magazines, not the work-free life. I am simply longing for more spaciousness in my calendar. When I am able to pause, take a step back, and examine my thoughts and emotions objectively, the bigger picture emerges with clarity. (This is one of the skills we are honing when we sit down each day to meditate. The more we practice noticing those thoughts, the more we can impartially observe them in the midst of our days.) With this bit of curious investigation and acceptance, the potentially destructive green-eyed monster skulks away as our focus turns to reality instead of assumptions, solutions instead of resentments.

It is only in naming our internal dialogue and feelings that allows us to tame them. (*Name it to tame it*, teaches the wise Dr. Dan Siegel.) Once I have acknowledged the existence of my thoughts and feelings, however unwelcome and humbling, I am free to choose what to do with them. Without the recognition of and owning up to my less-than-admirable musings, however, the potential for a palpable rift between my friend and me is likely, as envy positions itself firmly between the two of us, allowing those feelings of jealousy and resentment to fester.

This brief pause to gain a wider perspective not only alerts me to the green-eyed monster, but also reminds me that the proverbial grass is not always so green, opening up the perfect opportunity to reconnect with *why* I work (besides the financial need) and why I've opted for this particular career. Helping others is one of my most deeply held values. Though there are costs involved, I continue to *choose* my work because it brings me deep satisfaction. The thought of its absence is much too big a void, both in its lack of purpose and engagement and in the knowledge that without it I could imagine myself slipping easily into lethargy, boredom, and discontent. The benefits far outweigh the costs.

It is imperative not to compare the downsides of our lives to the perceived upsides of someone else's. Comparisons are unhelpful at best, downright disastrous at worst. Life happens to everyone; we all face daunting challenges at some point. Letting go of comparing allows me to return to the true source of my envy in the first place—the imbalance, the longing, the simple desire for more white space on my calendar. Instead, I can put some problem-solving skills to work: *How can I act on this realization? Where, precisely, can I carve out a bit of downtime and sense of freedom?*

Since that morning in the driveway I have been more conscious about taking slow, mindful walks in the sunshine and periodically shutting down the computer a bit early to simply sit and allow my mind to wander. Not only have I carved out a bit of white space in my calendar, but, just as important, I have reconnected with and strengthened my deeper motivations for choosing my particular career path. I harbor no great delusions, though, that I am free of the green-eyed monster's return. He will be back, I am sure. I will be waiting and curious to see what I can learn.

The Green-Eyed Monster Mindful Break

1 When you notice a twinge (or more like a punch in the gut) of envy, congratulate yourself for catching and owning this very human reaction, perhaps even thanking it for bringing such valuable information to light. Only when we are aware can we choose our response.

2 Pause to consider what the green-eyed monster is hoping to communicate. Sometimes the first answer is not the most enlightening. Keep asking. For instance, it may initially appear we are jealous of someone's wealth, but when examined more deeply, we might uncover our true longing for financial security, less worry, or more positive social regard.

3 Let go of comparing yourself with others, as this is essentially juxtaposing the outside of someone else with the inside of ourselves. Our comparisons are not exactly fair or accurate and bound to be a fruitless exercise in frustration. Firmly but kindly coax the focus back to yourself, heaping on a healthy dose of self-compassion and positive self-talk.

4 Take some action on your own behalf. You have bravely identified what it is you are craving; now what steps will you take to ameliorate it? What is the smallest, most easily accomplished move you can make toward fulfilling your longing? Start with that. If you find yourself stumped, check out the Make It Happen Mindful Break, page 217, for a little clarity.

5 Do not fear the green-eyed monster. He is a prevalent and, if handled skillfully, benevolent visitor to us all.

The U-Shaped Curve

Everything is figureoutable.   **—Marie Forleo**

Question: What's it like to be a published author?

    Answer: How long do you have?

1. Awesome.

2. Somewhat like bringing a baby into the world.[27]

3. The book-creating process is summed up perfectly by Adam Grant, *The New York Times*–bestselling author, professor, and motivation/meaning expert, in his popular TED talk.[28] In it, he asserts that the trajectory of any creative project resembles something like this:

This is awesome.

This is tricky.

This is crap.

I am crap.

This might be OK.

This is awesome.

That just about covers it—an accurate description of what writing books has felt like for me. This framework can also be applied to any longer-term task requiring innovation and persistence. By recognizing the pattern and anticipating the first few crappy drafts, we acknowledge and move past the "I am crap" stage without getting stuck there or abandoning ship completely. When we learn to expect this line of thinking, along with inevitable doubt and insecurity, we can invite it to have a seat right alongside us as we continue plugging away. In this way, we shift what Grant calls *self-doubt,* which can be paralyzing, to *idea-doubt,* which can be motivating. With idea-doubt, we can test out our creations and concepts without personalizing or internalizing their potential failings and pitfalls. Our creative projects are not us; they are fascinating U-shaped curve phenomena. Provided enough time, effort, and persistence, we will eventually land at the top of the ascending arc: "This is awesome!"

> *What I had that others didn't was a capacity for sticking to it.*
>
> —Doris Lessing

> *In the early and middle stages of any quest, there is often a Valley of Disappointment.*
>
> —James Clear

The U-Shaped Curve Mindful Break

❶ As you embark on any type of project, creative or otherwise, anticipate the strong likelihood of the U-shaped curve.

❷ When you find yourself frustrated, doubting your abilities, or about to give up, take a look at the curve and identify which step you are currently occupying. Congratulate yourself—you are right on track (though it might not feel so wonderful at the moment).

❸ You might benefit from stepping away for a short time, returning with fresh eyes, a usefully altered perspective, and a renewed sense of engagement.

❹ Whatever you do, though, be sure to come back, dive in once more, and allow yourself the delicious opportunity to reach the well-earned sweet taste of "This is awesome!" success.

Life as Pie

The price of anything is the amount of life you exchange for it.
—Henry David Thoreau

I find it ironic that penning a mindfulness guide for busy women gravely impedes my ability to live a mindful life. As a second-time author, I hold no fairy-tale misconceptions of what is involved in writing a book and have more than willingly—and gratefully—plunged into this exciting endeavor.

I was not feeling so lighthearted recently, though, when the stark realization hit that the manuscript deadline was drawing uncomfortably near. My typically placid nighttime dreams started to swim with inescapable anxiety. You know the kind, from showing up completely unprepared to offer a keynote speech in front of hundreds (at least this time fully clothed, thank God) to attempting to trap the wild animals loose in the basement, including an adorable panda bear. (*What*, you haven't had this one?) I began to experience a persistent heaviness in my chest, as if the aforementioned panda had taken a seat upon it. Basically, I was freaking out. Feeling stretched too thin and stressed out much of the time, I realized that something needed to give. It was time to reconfigure my priorities in order to meet the current demands and responsibilities in my life.

At some juncture or another, we busy women reach a point when the overall balance is off. This may manifest as a general sense of work–life lopsidedness—accompanied by utter confusion as to what to change or where to begin. Or, perhaps, a painful awareness of exactly which specific priorities we long for— exercise, a leisurely dinner out with our partner, caring for elderly relatives, or visiting a winery with friends—but deem impossible to incorporate into the fabric of our lives. As the numerous seasons of our life fluctuate, so does the requirement to reassess what is of greatest importance to us and, therefore, the best use of our time.

Only so much of how we spend our daily twenty-four hours is under our control, though it's likely more than we think. Caught up in the long-held habits and minutiae, it's easy to lose sight of the fact that some of our time can be deliberately manipulated to allow for more of what we crave. That is where the Life as Pie Mindful Break comes in. Conceptualizing those sixteen or so waking hours as composing a whole pie, we can intentionally slice and dice our life priority pieces (think: work, family, chores, and hobbies) to better suit our reality.

I love to play outside—hiking, biking, kayaking, running, and Rollerblading (against my better middle-aged judgment). There have been seasons in my life when all feels quite balanced, when the slice of pie devoted to hobbies is in abundance, the pace feels just right, and my engagement with life fulfilling. Other times, though, it feels like I am struggling desperately to keep my head above water (see Drowning in Chocolate Mindful Break page 103), and the hobby slice of pie dwindles to nearly nothing. This is a clue that the equilibrium is precariously askew.

On the flip side are those brief stretches of time when I feel a bit lost, with almost too much open space in my life pie. This showed up a few months after *Breathe, Mama, Breathe* was published. After the frantic publicity pace had subsided I was left adrift, wondering, *Now what?* For the most part, though, I am someone who tends to *overfill* my plate rather than be at a loss for what to place on it. Whatever the circumstances, I strive to carve out time for play and to keep the pieces of my pie as healthily proportional as possible.

As my manuscript deadline draws near, I have intentionally streamlined my life pie into one comprising primarily writing, psychotherapy, and family, with small slivers of self-care and miscellaneous mandatory obligations thrown in. A few of the additional cherished pieces are, for the time being, deliberately crowded out. I simultaneously hang on to the assurance, though, that when, breathing a huge sigh of relief, I e-mail these earnestly crafted sixty thousand words to my beloved editor a few months from now, the pieces temporarily put on hold will find their proper place in my life pie once again.

The Life as Pie Mindful Break

❶ On a piece of paper, pencil two large, equal-size circles side by side. The first is your current pie, the second, your ideal.

❷ In the current circle, divide up the general areas of your life into pie pieces according to how much time you now typically spend with each over the course of a week. Areas might include parenting/children, partners, family, friends/socializing, exercise, recreation/play/creativity, community, spirituality, education, work/career.

❸ In your ideal circle, divide up the areas into your optimal life pie. If doubt arises about the impossibility of your ideal, simply note those limiting beliefs and set them aside for now. This is purely a time to brainstorm and dream, without deep consideration of perceived barriers.

❹ Consider the two circles juxtaposed. What is prominent? What surprises you? What do you wish you had more time for? The ideal pie is a visual guide focusing on those areas we would like to modify. Note that this is an *ideal*, and some pieces may not be adjustable. If so, merciful acknowledgment and acceptance allows us to expend our precious energy on what *is* currently changeable.

❺ If your two pies are similar, they may require only tweaking in a few areas. If they appear quite unalike, it may at first seem inconceivable to maneuver from one to the other. Remember, where we place our attention and effort now affects the next moment in a sort of domino effect. Just one or two tiny adjustments at a time will get you to where you would eventually like to be.

6 Start with a single pie piece, choosing one aspect on which to focus. Take care not to overwhelm yourself. Regard it as an experiment or a challenge. You can begin with either an area you would like to expand or one you would like to diminish in size. For example, you may decide to reduce time spent on social media or scrolling through your phone. Keeping your ideal pie in mind, be deliberate in the amount of time allotted, say forty-five minutes each day, setting a timer if needed.

7 Now identify what you would like to add (either an entire pie slice or a single component within an existing pie piece) with that bit of newfound time—exercise, reading, spending time with friends, or some restful downtime?

8 Congratulate yourself as you fine-tune one area. Each mindful, positive change is steering you in the direction fitting for you. Revisit this mindful break every few weeks to hold yourself accountable. Observe and revel in the visual representation of your progress.

Disclaimer: Actual pie not included. I do love me some pie, though. After this mindful break, feel free to grab a generous slice of pie IRL and savor your delicious treat with the Lunch Mindful Break, page 89.

Play Hooky

I was becoming ill entirely too often. Nothing serious, just virus after virus, after overall exhaustion and malaise. Clearly, my immune system was operating suboptimally but I wasn't sure why. For the most part, I eat a fairly balanced, healthy diet; I exercise, meditate, take my vitamins, and wash my hands often. After months of this bothersome losing battle with germs, it was time for a comprehensive physical to delve further into what I might be missing. In order to rule out various possible contributing factors, I subjected myself to a thorough blood panel, home sleep study, and immune function tests, all of which were happily within normal limits.

At the rheumatologist visit to discuss results, I found myself seated across from the kind, fatherly physician whom I was meeting for the first time. As we dove into the discussion of my blood work and chronic symptoms, I was struck by how intently he listened while asking a number of probing questions into the structure and responsibilities of my life. Typically, when I slide into the role of patient it feels a bit foreign because, as a therapist, I am accustomed to focusing solely on the concerns of my client. Within a matter of minutes, though, I felt not only completely heard, valued, and seen, but choked up and touched at this rare moment of sincere compassion. Meeting my gaze, this thoughtful doctor said something that stopped me in my tracks: "You're doing much more than most people, you know."

"What? Really?" I uttered, stunned. I paused to ponder this. Though I do have a lot on my plate, I also consider myself to be just one among countless women with full lives, juggling many responsibilities, for the most part content and willing. Thankfully, I also have an equitable partner in my husband, whose days are just as packed as mine. I never deemed myself an outlier in this regard. "Yes, really. You have your own business, a busy family life, and are helping with your parents," he said.

Hold on, I thought, *I teach mindful balance, self-care, and healthy lifestyles. Do I seriously hold higher expectations for myself than for others?* Further self-inventory ensued. If I were a cartoon character my face would have worn a perplexed look while this thought bubble spontaneously appeared above my head. *Let's see . . . After years of ongoing child-related sleep interruptions, I have finally, consistently been sleeping through the night (mostly) for the past year or so. Though I am working hard to get seven hours of sleep a night, eat well, exercise, and meditate,*

I have also recently written, published, and diligently promoted a book, which causes me to step out of my comfort zone on a regular basis. On the home front, I am routinely mediating evolving conflict between my husband and teenaged daughter. I work full time with half-time childcare for my preschooler, which means squeezing in e-mails and phone calls at random hours of the day. I clean my own house, take care of my own psychotherapy administrative tasks, manage the complicated family schedule, and recently have been assisting more with Mom and Dad.

A few months earlier, I had found myself smack-dab in the sandwich generation as my parents were struggling with health issues. Infinitely grateful for such loving, giving parents, I more than willingly returned the favor. Although fully conscious of the increased worry and responsibilities, in the midst of it all, I merely shifted into survival mode, keeping my head down while attending to whatever was needed. *OK, agreed,* I conceded in the aforementioned thought bubble, *it has been a stressful patch.*

It's not that I was complaining, yearning for kudos, or feeling sorry for myself. Quite the opposite. I loved most of what I was doing. I chose it and looked around at my little world, grateful, on a regular basis. I simply took for granted that I could manage all that my life entailed. It had never occurred to me that I might have been expecting too much of my physical and emotional reserves.

I was reminded that life needn't necessarily feel *bad* for it to be *too much,* for the necessity of spending a little more time on rest, on slowing down, on whatever nourishes our souls. Otherwise, we are left plodding through the days, the months, the years, in this automatic, semiconscious way, attending to others and infinite life requirements, without turning the focus back on ourselves to assess what it is we really hunger for at the most basic level.

You know what else this kindhearted physician helped me realize I needed? *Permission to play hooky.* Permission (from myself) to take a brief respite from my own business (you'd think, as the boss, doing so wouldn't be so guilt inducing—and you'd be wrong), from my family, from my life. This felt rebellious, immediately taking me back to my high school years, when, as a conscientious and overscheduled teen, my parents allowed me to play hooky, savoring a mental health day without the need to first drive myself to exhaustion and illness. I can still wistfully recall the delicious feeling of rest and quiet as the world continued on for the day without me. I couldn't go out of the house lest my benign deceit was discovered, so I blissfully sat home reading, consuming mindless TV, recharging my body and mind.

Perhaps you've never played hooky a day in your life and this sounds outrageous or irresponsible. Maybe your parents would never have allowed such a thing, requiring you to be on your deathbed before any school could be missed. Whatever your previous experience with sick days, I'll let you in on a little secret: *You are now a grown-ass woman who can make her own choices. Even if you are the boss, you can take the day off when you are not really sick.* (I am emphasizing this to myself as well as to you.)

I highly recommend (to us both) a full-on mental health "sick" day. Though the vast majority of the mindful breaks in this book are brief and meant to be incorporated in the midst of the day, the Play Hooky Mindful Break is unique in that I am advocating strongly for an entire planned day off. A day to play hooky from work, from responsibilities, from your life. Some of you will say this is impossible and maybe—*maybe*—this is true. This break can last anywhere from a few short minutes to an entire, legitimate day off—or any length of time you can muster.

The Play Hooky Mindful Break

❶ Get quiet, take a few moments, and dream a little. If I were to grant you one whole day when you could jump off the spinning world and do whatever your little heart desired, how, and with whom, would you spend it? Would it be a wild adventure à la *Ferris Bueller's Day Off*? Would you lie in bed under the covers with Netflix, Ben, and Jerry? Would you pull on your running shoes and head out into the woods solo, or with your partner or loyal dog in tow? Maybe you'd grab your girlfriend, splurge on an hour massage and mani-pedi with dinner and wine to follow. Listen in on what your soul is craving without throwing up the barriers just yet.

❷ Can you schedule a day off? Before you shout *No way!* consider that the world will not come crashing down if you miss one single day of work. Of course, you'll want to do this responsibly, we don't want a (*Bueller . . . Bueller*) unexcused absence to ensue. I trust you know the ins and outs of your particular workplace—whether a day scheduled off in advance is a necessity or if your position allows for a more last-minute day to play hooky on a whim.

❸ Notice the reasons your mind concocts as to why this is not feasible and assess their true validity. If a full day is not in the cards right now, schedule a few hours. Maybe leave your office and go for a picnic lunch or spend a few minutes window-shopping, taking in the sights. Even a half-hour mini respite can feel wonderfully decadent.

❹ If and when thoughts of guilt arise, acknowledge them, brush them gently aside, and remind yourself of our universal deep-seated need for self-care and rest, so rare and fleeting. You will return to work rejuvenated, a boon to any workplace. Treat yourself with the same care that kindly doctor showed me. Each of us, by nature of being human, is deserving. Why not you?

Anchoring (for Challenging Moments)

———

Though there are seasons of life in which we contentedly coast, inevitably, a circumstance (or confluence of them) occurs that, like a powerful tidal wave, threatens to knock us off our feet. The human condition is such that we are often caught off guard when our turn arrives. So it was for me with my father's cancer diagnosis and progressively declining health.

After he lived with terminal cancer for a number of months, the time to say a final goodbye to my beloved dad drew near. I spent hours sitting at the edge of his hospital bed, holding his hand, watching him sleep, allowing my thoughts to drift and my emotions to rise, taking in the quiet, witnessing the rising and falling of his barrel-like rib cage, placing my hand gently over his heart.

Inhale, exhale. Rising, falling. Let go, let go. . . .

As I sat drinking in the connection, I was swiftly transported back to the birth of my son nearly a decade before, when—after a tumultuous pregnancy, in the quiet of the hospital night—I sat for hours gazing at the beautiful, wizened face of my healthy newborn, in awe of each rise and fall of his small but mighty chest.

Inhale, exhale. Rising, falling. Welcome, welcome. (Thank you, thank you.)

Days later, as I sat down to write about my dad's passing, it occurred to me that our long goodbye was a joint sacred meditation of sorts. I have no doubt my mindfulness practice supported my ability to sit, stay, and feel deeply.

The seasons of life are ever-evolving. Throughout the seasons, the breath remains constant, anchoring us, calming us, helping us through intense grief, love, awe, and joy. Connecting to the breath allows us to bear gut-wrenching emotion without drowning in it, to integrate our experiences, and to head out into the world more vulnerable and raw—yet more compassionate and profoundly changed.

There are seasons in life when we push and grow, purposefully living full-out and immersed. Other seasons call for radical slowing down, perhaps even screeching to a swift halt, simply to be, feel, and take in what life has brought our way. This is not so easy, of course, but wholly worthwhile and empowering in the compassionate, gritty resilience it creates.

Leaning in heavily to the mindfulness tools I have practiced over the years allowed me to physically sit with the emotionally loaded thoughts and memories as I grieved my dad. I let the tears flow when the lump in my throat arrived. I did my best to sleep when the exhaustion hit. I laughed heartily with wet eyes when recalling a sweet memory. I noticed my energy return as the seasons turned and once again I shifted my gaze outward into the life that calls to me to engage, love, teach, and learn.

This is the strength of mindful empowerment in action and why I am on a mission to share it with you. Human suffering is universal; no one is immune. I hope this mindful break serves as a helpful conduit to feel life deeply—and as a reassuring lifeline to keep you planted on solid emotional ground.

Inhale, exhale. Rising, falling. Grateful, humble, strong.

The Anchoring Mindful Break

Stay in the moment.
We can often tolerate more than we first realize. If we can bring a sense of openness, curiosity, and courage to the situation, we reap the rewards of experiencing life more fully.

Rest in the breath.
There are times when the breath is enough to anchor us. Attention to the inhale and exhale is sufficient, to help us ride the waves of intensity.

Just as in meditation, repeatedly return the attention to the breath each time it wanders, alternating with noticing body sensations, if helpful.

Choose a soothing mantra or phrase.
Place your hands to your heart. What reassuring message do you need to hear most right now? It can be as simple as *I'm okay, I'm safe,* or *I can do this.*

When it feels like too much

There is no medal for bravery when we are bowled over by life. If the moment feels too intense, do not force yourself to remain in it.

When flooded with emotion, simply noticing the breath may be too overwhelming or even counterproductive. Here are a few other ways to ride out the emotional storm until you are on solid footing once again.

Connect with the five senses.

Look up and around for five things you can see, four you can touch, three you can hear, two you can smell, and one you can taste. Don't get caught up in the exact order. This can also be as simple as noticing three blue items in the room. Intentionally observing our senses serves as a helpful distraction from overwhelm, by grounding us in our outer world.

Get grounded.

Notice how the feet are supported by the floor and bring your full attention there. What sensations do you notice? Warmth, coolness, moisture, tingling? Can you sense your socks, shoes, or bare feet on the floor?

Home in on body sensations.

With both hands, lightly tap the arms, legs, stomach, or cheeks. Stand up and shake it out. Give yourself a big hug and notice the sensations as you gently squeeze up and down your arms.

Keep it subtle.
If others are around and you're searching for a nonobvious way to quietly ground yourself, place your palms together in your lap. Tap each finger together once, beginning with the thumbs and progressively moving through the rest. Come back to the thumbs and tap them together twice, and so on. You can complete five rounds or stop when you feel sufficiently calm.

What do you need?
Once you feel reasonably grounded and calm, ask yourself what you need next. Research shows that women often crave the company of others in challenging emotional times, which is referred to as the tend-and-befriend instinct. Call a friend, text for a bit, or ask someone to simply sit quietly alongside you. Go for a walk outside, soak in the tub, nap, or even run it out. Indulge in a long, ugly cry; journal; scream into a pillow; or give yourself a big, soothing bear hug. Ultimately, you know yourself well. Whatever you need is fine. Now is exactly the time to ask for it.

Benevolent Badass Boundaries

—

Just when I thought I pretty much had this healthy boundary thing nailed down, a message from a woman I respect proved otherwise. Nikki's email popped into my inbox on one of those weeks when, despite my best intentions, my cup overfloweth. I was feeling burned out from giving three talks *about burnout* over the course of a few days. In addition to my week of temporarily burning out on burnout, meeting with therapy clients, and recording podcasts, I was also knee-deep in the process of creating a brand-new program.

As a coach looking to expand her business, Nikki asked if I would be up for a call to talk about how she might gain local media exposure to reach her audience and share her message. Though I was overwhelmed and decidedly did not want to add another thing to my plate, I wrestled with saying no to someone I really wanted to help. So I did what I always do when faced with a dilemma—no matter how small. I did . . . nothing.

Huh? Yes, nothing for a day or so. I set the decision aside; I slept on it. When I came back to revisit it, my answer felt the same, even clearer. *I need to focus on my priorities right now. I need to say NO to everything else so I can say YES to what I am creating.*

I wrote back to Nikki, doing my best to decline gracefully, hoping she would understand, feeling slightly uncomfortable yet confident in my stance. I shared my current focus and a few brief media tips, promising a forthcoming public blog post with more information. And guess what? Nikki wrote back, telling me how much she respected my healthy boundaries (which, of course, spoke to her own), thereby kindly supporting another woman in pursuit of her goals.

Ultimately, we can't go about the business of reclaiming our time, energy, and purpose without a deep consideration of boundaries. Boundaries help us set limits, demarcating where we end and where our responsibilities to others begin. Physical boundaries consist of material items, our bodies, and our surroundings. Mental boundaries comprise our emotions, thoughts, and time.

Many of us are comfortable with setting boundaries on behalf of others (our kids, partners, or close friends) yet are plagued with guilt and self-criticism when establishing our own. However uncomfortable we may initially feel, when we clarify our boundaries and protect them, everyone wins. We not only communicate categorically what we will and will not tolerate, we also model for those around us how it can be done with both mutual respect and grace.

The Benevolent Badass Boundaries Mindful Break

Notice when you may be compromising your boundaries. Are you sighing, automatically resigned to a habitual sense of obligation, or, perhaps, silently screaming NO! while outwardly nodding SURE! out of that old nice-girl habit? Signs range from subtle to impossible-to-ignore. You might experience tension in the shoulders, jaw, and stomach or an overall tired, drained sensation. Emotions of frustration, anger, or resentment may arise.

Offer the benefit of the doubt. Take a deep breath and remind yourself that though a few folks may be fully aware of the sizable burden of their request, most would be dismayed to know they were inducing hardship.

Determine whether this situation requires setting a boundary. If not completely evident (and whenever possible), employ the twenty-four-hour waiting period before committing. If, after some time, the signals feel just as strong, it is time for benevolent badass boundary-setting. On to the next step.

Get clear and shore up strength. How do you want the new boundary to look? Is there a compromise, or is a hard NO necessary? How will you know when the boundary is in alignment and working for you? For example, your body might feel relaxed. You might once again feel in control of your time, energy, and surroundings. Stand strong and repeat after me: *I have every right to create and hold healthy boundaries.*

Set it. Communicate clearly and *without apology* about the specifics of this boundary. You may or may not want to share your reasons—you do not owe anyone an explanation. Practice on a trusted friend first, if needed. Keep it short and simple. There is always the chance, of course, that you will be met with resistance or that the other person will attempt to—consciously or not—steamroll right over your carefully constructed boundaries. That is their issue, not yours. If this is an important boundary, do not back down, however uncomfortable and unfamiliar that is to you. If you are not in the habit of practicing assertiveness—using your voice with firm kindness—it can seem downright aggressive at first. It grows much easier over time.

Celebrate! You will be amazed at how often others graciously accept your boundaries. Though you may experience some residual guilt and self-doubt, take note of your body sensations, emotions, and thoughts. Is there a palpable sense of relief? Pride? Empowerment? Offer yourself a well-deserved high-five for taking care of and prioritizing yourself.

Your Personal Board
of Advisors

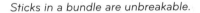

Sticks in a bundle are unbreakable.

—Kenyan proverb

My mom is my greatest champion. So much so, in fact, that for years we have lovingly compared her enthusiastic praise to a scene in Eddie Murphy's *The Nutty Professor*, in which the grandma, lauding her grandson's simple accomplishment, springs up and down in her chair with unbridled excitement, clapping, and shouting, *Hercules! Hercules!* As a fanatical supporter, my mom may not be my most objective source of feedback. Instead, as a member of my Personal Board of Advisors, her strength lies in her natural capacity to buoy me up rather than telling it to me straight.

We can all profit from developing our own Personal Board of Advisors—for advice, accountability, honest feedback, deeper work relationships, and to remind us that we are not alone in our struggles. Our board can support our value-driven career and partake in the celebration of ongoing success.

Women often subscribe to the idea of a false promise of meritocracy; that is, in order to prove ourselves and progress in our careers, we must put our heads down, remain consistently task focused, work longer and harder than our male counterparts. What falls to the wayside, though, is the development of meaningful, mutually beneficial relationships that are just as vital to our well-being and growth. With the intentional establishment of our Personal Board of Advisors, the cultivation of connection and relationship development regain their rightful place among our top priorities.

Set your life on fire. Seek those who fan your flames.

—Rumi

Though requiring a bit more effort and time, there is more power in groups than in going solo. With a deliberate attitude of support and mutual respect, the sum total of awesomeness is much greater than its parts. Throw a diverse group of women together in a safe, open environment and unpredictable magic happens. Seek out those women with whom you can be vulnerable, real, and balanced. Start the process of creating your own Personal Board of Advisors today.

Your Personal Board of Advisors Mindful Break

1 Name those already on your team, regardless of whether you have ever considered your own board of advisors. Most likely there is at least one currently sitting member whom you can count on.

❷ If you have a hardy circle, determine if you would like to broaden your board.

❸ Identify the specific strengths that each existing member brings. For instance, honesty, strong work ethic, fiscal knowledge, managerial experience, sense of humor, ability to consider the big picture. The uncompromising requirement is that she have your best interest at heart.

❹ What qualities are you still searching for in your members? Though your board should consist of women IRL, it might first help to bring to mind a few inspirational women you admire (in person or from afar) and why, in order to identity who might be the best fit. For example, I respect Michele Obama for her intelligence, work ethic, physical and character strength, and commitment to use her social influence for good, so I might seek out someone with a few of those attributes.

❺ Name two steps you can take toward building your board. Schedule those into your calendar this week.

❻ In what ways, exactly, are you hoping your board members can assist you? Time management? Conflict resolution? Connecting with others? General mentorship?

❼ Remember these relationships are a two-way street. Be on the lookout for ways to reciprocate. It may take time and patience to find and grow those relationships. Focus as best you can on process, rather than outcome.

❽ Finally, it never hurts to have a designated Personal Board of Advisors champion, right Mom? *Hercules!*

Gas Pedal or Brake

One icy winter weekend found me prone on the couch, unhappily under the weather and a generous heap of blankets. A modest pile of books and a warm mug of lemon ginger tea rested on the coffee table next to me. Despite an overall unpleasant malaise, it also felt *freaking amazing* to fully succumb to a rare mode of hibernation.

Can you hear the undercurrent of guilt in my admission? Yes, despite imploring others to lay off the accelerator and instead lay flat out on their couches for periodic, routine R&R, I often wrestle with offering myself said permission. I've come to realize that, for me, the guilt arises not so much from societal Superwoman expectations as it does from the always-lurking suspicion that if I use the day to stop and regroup, I will sorely regret it *tomorrow* as once again I come face-to-face with that interminable to-do list. In other words, if I *play* (or rest) today, I will certainly *pay* tomorrow. Not exactly the relaxing mindset to which I aspire. (I'm in need of these mindful breaks just as much as you!)

Whether borne of time scarcity, internalized expectations, or any other source, offering ourselves permission to rest is a challenging universal theme. We are doers, movers, and shakers. And whether consciously or not, we are habituated to the feel of our foot on the gas pedal—even *addicted to* the rush—and loathe to resist the constant craving for more.

Of course, we can all agree that, objectively, it is not ideal to pump the brakes on our speedy pace of life *only* when we fall ill or when some other life event suddenly throws the emergency brake on *for us*. Despite my own occasional resistance, I am all about the very real necessity for rest, recuperation, and temporary setting-aside of the infinite to-do list. There are days, weeks, even seasons of life that call for coasting, easing up on the accelerator of life.

Yes, we all benefit from intervals of slowing down—either easing up on the gas or applying gentle pressure to the brake. Appreciating the moment, periodically reflecting on all we've already accomplished, abandoning the notion that we are continuous improvement projects rather than human beings—all are essential when you *Don't Forget to Breathe*.

Lately, I've been encountering a dramatic shift in the media sphere that takes this self-care imperative even further: An anti-hustle, anti-ambition, anti-striving culture is slowly taking shape in the realm of work–life balance. The overarching message: *STOP. We should ALL be slamming on the brakes indefinitely, giving ourselves a collective break at life. You are good enough just as you are. Let go of striving; there is nothing wrong with you. There is zero need to grind, to continually prove yourself.*

To this, I take exception. The underlying anti-hustle assumption is that the sole source of our ambition is our insecurities—that all driven, goal-achieving women are unconsciously caught in the throes of never-good-enough-itis. Though this may be true at times, the desire for self-improvement is certainly not always rooted in this deficient core belief.

As wise women, we know that inextricably equating self-worth purely with our numerous accomplishments and accolades is un- and counterproductive. We are fully aware that *who we are* as women, how we treat others, and our unique personal qualities—that's the stuff.

Do we get tripped up by it at times? Absolutely. We can all fall off-course occasionally (hence the need for this book). Yet so many of us are playing big *for the thrill of it*. It's fun, challenging, and keeps life interesting. Applying consistent, firm pressure to the brake pedal for the rest of our lives, like the new anti-hustler movement recommends? No way. How uninspiring, depressing, and, well, flat-out boring.

As much as I understand the impulse to do so (we have been, after all, surviving a pandemic and plenty other upheavals), *let's not* completely acquiesce to a permanent state of hibernation. *We women* not only deserve more, the world also deserves our unique gifts, talents, and personalities. Growth and striving, when carried out with intention and awareness, lights us up, infusing our surroundings with contagious energy and possibility. Self-care, after all, is not *always* about resting.

Inevitably, it comes back to balance: knowing when to ease up on the gas and when to accelerate, when to apply slow pressure to the brakes, and when life might require that trusty emergency brake.

When we are ready to achieve, we can make sure we are hustling with intention, balancing the ambition, and going after what we *really want* rather than what we believe is expected of us. We can also be grateful, content, and happy in the process.

The Gas Pedal or Brake Mindful Break will serve us over our lifetime—myself included. Now excuse me as I ready my books, tea, and blankets for a blissful hour of hibernation mode. It's time for a brief deceleration before I'm back in the driver's seat, rejuvenated and ready to embrace forward momentum and, quite possibly, a bit of speed.

The Gas Pedal or Brake Mindful Break

1. Pause and assess your speed.

Are you tired? Burned out? Sighing a lot? Wistfully wishing you could crawl under the covers and hibernate for an entire week? Sounds like you could benefit from pumping the brakes. What is not absolutely necessary in your schedule or on your to-do list? Remove it, cancel it, or postpone it, if possible. Look ahead and schedule some open space in your calendar when *you must* rest and slow down.

Are you feeling bored? Uninspired? Struggling with

motivation or movement? This typically calls for some pressure on the gas pedal. It might be time for an engaging hobby, new side hustle, or out-of-your-comfort-zone work project. Take heed, though; burnout can also mimic boredom. Make sure to ask yourself, *What do I really need at this time?* Then, please listen and act accordingly.

Ultimately, we want to head in the direction that lights us up without burning us out. Periodically pause and assess—then speed up or slow down as necessary along the way.

2. What's driving the striving?

What is the underlying motivation for your ambition? Is it rooted in fear and scarcity or growth and challenge?

Fear sounds like your inner critic: negative, perfectionistic, self-doubting, insecure. This fear might arise from an internal thought or external pressure. Does it sound like *I want to* or *I have to/should*? If so, it's time to hit the brakes.

Healthy ambition and growth may feel exciting, energizing, and a little scary, while causing you to unconsciously lean in with your curiosity piqued. Gas pedal, it is! Go for it and enjoy!

3. Ditch the guilt.

When it comes to offering yourself permission to rest, you may feel guilt. Notice it, acknowledge it, then anchor yourself in what you need. Over time and with some practice, when you get quiet and take a moment to dig deep, you will know what is called for. Guilt be damned.

Beginner's Mind

—

My destination is no longer a place, rather a new way of seeing.
—Marcel Proust

One of my favorite things about having kids is viewing the world afresh through their eyes. When my son was four and entering into that endearing, nonstop talking, curious-about-the-world phase, he posed the question of how babies in the womb receive nourishment. After listening to my best attempt at an age-appropriate explanation, he pondered the information for a moment, then recapped, "So let me get this straight. You ate food, it went into *your* belly, then into *my* belly button through your *extension cord*?"

I paused a beat as my love for him grew impossibly greater. I didn't have the heart to correct that perfectly mistaken word choice. "Extension cord. Exactly," I replied, "and there has been an invisible extension cord connecting our hearts ever since."

I imagine in the future the poor kid will fail that portion of the anatomy test, but for now I couldn't help but savor the innocently bungled terminology. (Seriously, don't you think extension cord is a more apt description than umbilical? Latin, schmatin.)

Zen Buddhists refer to this fresh perspective-taking as *beginner's mind,* much like viewing the world through the eyes of a child. With the help of my little guy I had now shifted my perspective from taking the world for granted into beginner's mind. How lovely and amazing and, get this, totally applicable at work.

This is a wonderful day. I've never seen this one before.

—Maya Angelou

We (ahem) older folks can cultivate this childlike sense of awe and curiosity in our lives as well. Fortunately, we don't always need a little one around to assist us. This mindful break is all about integrating beginner's mind into our days, as boredom, complacency, and disregard cannot coexist with genuine interest and wonder. Instead, we can choose awe, appreciation, and awareness. Doing so helps us feel younger and has been shown to literally slow the aging process as well. By moving through our days with intention, we become aware of what is so often overlooked or dismissed out of hand.

Beginner's Mind Mindful Break

Choose one activity, at work or at home, to apply beginner's mind. Imagine you have never encountered this situation before. What do you notice? What is most prevalent? How does this impact or shift the moment for you?

Your thoughts will likely wander off on a tangent as you play with this mindful break. Bring a curious attitude and, without judgment, turn your attention back to the task at hand. Repeat as necessary.

Experiment with applying beginner's mind to all sorts of activities, from driving to e-mailing to sitting through that afternoon meeting. When we bring beginner's mind to everyday mundane or rote tasks, we are not only granted a fresh perspective; we will consequently reach our goals with less resistance or frustration.

Go ahead, allow yourself to savor a taste of that child-like fascination with life—both at work and out in the big, wide-open world. It's yours for the taking.

What Gnaws at You?

—

Our callings challenge us to view our pain about the world differently—not as something uncomfortable to turn away from but as an indicator of the brokenness we're meant to help repair.

—Tara Mohr

Sometimes we witness something so disturbing it is forever burned into our memory, gnawing at us for days, months, or years after. When interviewing human rights advocate Khine Zaw she shared with me one such encounter. While working as an advocate in Thailand, Khine encountered a nine-year-old Burmese girl who was being prostituted by her own family. Khine was powerless to save her, and the little girl's devastating predicament never left her mind. From that tragically planted seed years ago, Khine has since grown a business devoted to supporting and empowering female survivors of trauma.

At other times we might be haunted by missed opportunities or a sense of emptiness from not living up to our full potential.

After years of balancing full-time work with single motherhood, Jill was feeling stagnant and unfulfilled in her personal life. For as long as she could remember she had dreamed of being a stand-up comedian. Finding a local amateur event, she inked it into her calendar, spending hours writing and rewriting her eight-minute skit. Nervous, terrified, yet invigorated, Jill strutted up on that stage in front of her family, boyfriend, and teenage son. As she recounted the high she experienced from the laughter and applause, her pride and bliss were evident.

I am no longer accepting the things I cannot change. I am changing the things I cannot accept.
—Angela Davis

What Khine and Jill both shared was the nagging feeling of some unfinished business gnawing at them. When we carry around such haunting notions unattended to, they are bound to keep showing up repeatedly, unnecessarily consuming precious thought, energy, and emotion. What gnaws at us offers us information about how we might want to handle situations differently in the future, a wrong we need to right, or even a clue that points us in the direction of our deepest unfulfilled longings. Once we distill the message from what gnaws at us, we can go about the business of decluttering the baggage or transforming that yearning into a reality.

What Gnaws at You? Mindful Break

1 Pay attention to what haunts or harasses you. It may be an unpleasant experience, an unfulfilled aspiration from long ago, or even a conversation you wish you could change. What is the lesson, message, or longing found within?

2 Determine if this is an area you feel compelled to pursue. Take care to not be pulled into the common *I-am-just-one-person-what-can-I-alone-accomplish?* fallacy. If each of us acts on our beliefs, it adds up to significant change and personal fulfillment.

3 Applaud yourself for bravely recognizing and addressing what has been gnawing at you.

4 Identify one small action that you can take toward your dream or cause. That, my friend, is exactly where you need to begin.

Tame Your Inner Workaholic

Radical prioritization means recognizing that we are never going to solve the problem of having too much to do by shrinking the amount we have to do . . . but we can change how we think about what we have to do and how we engage with the process of prioritizing.

—Leah Weiss

I love to work. Is that weird? This did not happen by accident or sheer luck, as I deliberately created an engaging career by following my curiosity, digging in with persistence, untangling self-doubt from my true capabilities, and devoting time and chutzpah.

Not an extreme person by nature, I am more of the moderate, cautious sort. With writing, reading, and learning, however, I am *into it*. It excites me, energizes me, and gets my creative juices flowing. If not for my family and life responsibilities, I could easily live for days happily surrounded only by piles of books, assorted snacks, and a warm, cozy blanket. Regardless of how much I adore my family, there are moments when I am so in the flow of work that I fantasize briefly about an entire uninterrupted week to myself. It can be painful to wrestle myself away from the magnetic draw of meaningful work in order to maintain some semblance of balance as responsibility beckons. And, yes, there are certainly times that I, too, simply forget to breathe. Once I do shift gears and dive back into family life, spending time with them is, of course, wonderful, worthwhile, and fulfilling.

Some of us overwork to avoid facing unpleasant issues in our personal lives, some for financial survival or security, others to avoid negative job consequences. If we are fortunate enough, we work primarily for purpose and fulfillment. This, too, can become problematic—if taken to an unhealthy extreme. Working excessively negatively impacts our overall well-being, brings us to the edge of burnout, and also follows the law of diminishing returns: After a certain number of hours, our productivity declines significantly. There is such a thing as too much of a good thing. Moderation and balance are key. According to research, "If you work between thirty and fifty hours per week, adding more hours to the job lifts your performance. But once you're working between fifty and sixty-five hours per week, the benefit of adding additional hours drops off. And if you're working sixty-five hours or more, overall performance declines as you pile on the hours."[31] If you struggle with overdoing the work thing, it is important for your health and your productivity to dial it back. The Tame Your Inner Workaholic is here to do just that.

The Tame Your Inner Workaholic Mindful Break

① Recognize if this mindful break applies to you. Some of us are fully aware of our proclivity to dive headfirst into work, others not so much. If you are questioning your level of workaholic tendencies, chances are good you are a candidate. Is it difficult for you to stop when other life responsibilities call? Has someone close to you expressed frustration about the amount of time you work? Other clues come from within. When I am in overwork mode, I begin unconsciously sighing, deeply and frequently, or start to feel disconnected from family or friends.

② If you find yourself in this camp, know you are in good company and that there is no need to self-judge. Recognizing your penchant for overwork empowers you to modify it as you see fit. High five to you for owning it.

③ Kindly examine whether you are working to avoid a contentious home life or relationship, social anxiety, fear of being alone, or other stressor in your life. If this is the case, it may be time to mindfully, cautiously face what you have been avoiding. Talking to a friend or seeking out a therapist can help you sort through your avoidance, offering compassionate, more deliberate, alternatives.

④ If avoidance doesn't seem to fit the bill and you work too much for enjoyment and purpose, you are in a fortunate position, though you will still benefit from some tempering.

5 To tame your inner workaholic, let her know you understand it can be tough to pull herself away but that other parts of you need to encounter and savor life as well. Work can never replace relationships and experiences, regardless of how much we love it. If we have heeded that inner workaholic for years, we may need to reidentify how we like to spend our time and with whom. Experiment and have fun with this.

6 Pay attention to clues your body offers in order to gauge the best balance for you—tightness and tiredness indicate the balance is off; a sense of ease, lightness, and clearheadedness point to a healthy balance.

7 With kindness and nonjudgment, continue to transfer some weight back to the *life* side of your overall work-life balance.

Falling Off the Wagon

In the innovation space, compassion is at the heart of failing fast and recovering quickly.

—Monica Worline

After waking and shuffling to the bathroom this morning, I gazed in the mirror and recoiled a bit, taken aback by my reflection. The greenish-gray cast set below puffy, glazed-over eyes loudly announced the dull ache in my head. And though this unpleasant grogginess, reminiscent of a mild college-age hangover, did not originate in the over-imbibing of alcohol, I should not have been surprised.

You see, last night, returning home from work a little after 8:00 PM, hungry, tired, and spent from a full week, I sat down with a comforting bowl of pesto-tossed pasta and a glass of Old Vine Zin. Later, satisfied, relaxed, and sinking into the couch with a delightfully gratifying episode of my latest TV show, Ben & Jerry began whispering my name from the depths of the nearby freezer. *New York Super Fudge Chunk*, I'm fairly certain I heard, their familiar voices full of temptation. *Coming, my loves*, I answered silently, heaving myself off the couch. And the rest, my friend, is history.

Fortunately, for the most part, I prefer to live in the land of moderation and don't make a habit of 9:00 PM carb-loading followed by a glass of wine and generous bowl of ice cream. I am fully aware that I feel and operate at my best when I wake and go to bed early, meditate, exercise, eat reasonably healthy, and enjoy no more than a few glasses of wine a week. There are occasions, however (to which my sweet Ben & Jerry can attest), when the need arises for me to revisit the trusty old Falling Off the Wagon Mindful Break. This break speaks to the remorse, guilt, and self-judging experienced after falling back into old, unhealthy habits. It is about how to pick ourselves up, dust ourselves off, and get right back into healthy working order.

The Falling Off the Wagon Mindful Break

❶ Identify the conditions that contributed to your falling off of the wagon. Exhaustion, stress, relationship conflict, feelings of helplessness, and unfavorable self-talk are common negative internal influences. Others might include hanging out with a difficult person or engaging in an exhausting activity while minimizing or rationalizing your behavior.

❷ Recognize where the habit went off the rails and how to avoid that error in the future.

❸ Assess whether you attempted too much, too quickly and recalibrate the steps to meet your intentional goal as necessary. (See also Make It Happen, page 217.)

❹ Instead of self-judging, thank the Falling Off the Wagon consequences for the reminder as to why you established that new habit in the first place.

❺ Own it, take responsibility, and let go of the rehashing. We cannot change the past, even the very recent past. The best we can do is set up the conditions for success and continue to make intentional choices in each moment.

❻ Reconnect to the values that underpin this healthy habit. (See also Your Inner Compass, page 207.)

❼ Climb back up on that wagon and recommit to the habit. Onward and upward you go.